FIT AT
FIFTYSOMETHING

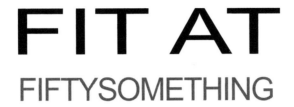

FIT AT
FIFTYSOMETHING

Brian F. Bolstad DMD

TWO HARBORS PRESS

Two Harbors Press
212 3rd Avenue North, Suite 290
Minneapolis, MN 55401
612.455.2293
www.TwoHarborsPress.com

ISBN - 978-1-935097-23-5
ISBN - 1-935097-23-7
LCCN - 2009929771

Book sales for North America and international:
Itasca Books, 3501 Highway 100 South, Suite 220
Minneapolis, MN 55416
Phone: 952.345.4488 (toll free 1.800.901.3480)
Fax: 952.920.0541; email to orders@itascabooks.com

Cover Design by Kristeen Wegner
Typeset by Peggy LeTrent

Printed in the United States of America

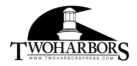

Contents

INTRODUCTION

You picked up this book, probably based on the title and cover, so I'll guess there is a good chance you are over forty and likely close to or past fifty. In this age range you have fewer days in front of you than behind you. That's not good, but then it's not entirely bad either. By now you have lived enough that you have probably acquired some degree of wisdom. Only the biggest of idiots and grandest of fools can pass through that many days and learn nothing. The fact that you are reading a book about self improvement by definition means you're not either. Rare is the human who gets much past forty and is not experiencing the diminution of faculties that comes with time. You can't turn on the TV without seeing advertisements aimed at ED, arthritis pain, insomnia, wrinkled skin, grey hair, osteoporosis, and vitamin deficiencies. Wall Street certainly has noticed you and is ready to sell you a variety of pills for whatever ails you. Don't get me wrong, every medication has its appropriate indicated use and genuine benefit. This is not a treatise on holistic herbal all-natural anything.

We're going to take a relatively comprehensive look at a multitude of areas that make up our lives. We'll ask a few questions and provide some relatively simple common sense answers based on sound medical science. And we are going to be brief. And we are going to do this on the cheap. You are not going to have to spend any significant number of dollars to get yourself on the right track. For a lot of people, coming up with the number of dollars it takes to pay for everything in your life is part of what keeps you stuck on the wrong track. In my time spent studying health issues I have come across some very detailed and thorough protocols and prescriptions for measuring your nutritional deficiencies, hormonal deficiencies coupled with one on one fitness training. These programs were always relatively expensive and out of reach for the average budget.

To start with, how do you feel? How do you want to feel? And what can you do to feel better? If the answers to the first two are "run down" and "good," then the rest of this book will answer the third. The primary underlying principle behind this book is showing you how to become truly physically fit. In the process, the goal is to make every day remaining in front of you as good as possible. After all, they are limited in number.

When you are young, you do because you can

When you are old, you can because you do

Doc

YOU ANIMAL YOU

You may not have thought about it much lately, but you really do have a lot in common with your dog. And your cat. And the robin outside your window. And the animals of the Rocky Mountains. In spite of your intellect, you are still an animal. Physically, biologically, biochemically, you're an animal. The last few hundred years have seen such a huge increase in technological advancement by humans that it is very easy to delude ourselves about the consequences of our behavior. Hunger has been all but eliminated in civilized societies. Medical care is widely available in Western societies. Few suffer from extremes of cold or heat, wind or rain. The condition of extremes of natural elements killing significant numbers of humans happens in only the most backward and repressive societies.

Humans evolved over the last 100,000 or so years. From that time up until about 1900, most humans led a very hand to mouth existence. Very few people earned a living performing some relatively sedentary task. Most applied their knowledge to some physically demanding endeavor, from hunting and gathering, as early man did from dawn to dusk, to woodworking, farming, etc., later on. In modern times most work involves service or information transfer. The point here, of course, is that for most of human history, if you did not perform some physically demanding task from dawn to dusk, there was a much higher chance you were going to suffer the pain of hunger. People were highly motivated to get off their asses. Lazy and sedentary behavior was rarely tolerated. If an individual was not constantly moving around in a productive manner he or she was less likely to obtain enough to eat, and therefore survive long enough to reproduce. The perfectly natural response to that is to feel like "I sure am glad I don't have to work that damn hard". The point being, the need for regular exercise probably runs much deeper in our genetic makeup than we are used to thinking. As omnivores, we humans share characteristics with both carnivores and herbivores.

A pack of wolves may hunt for weeks to succeed in a large kill, such as an elk. During that time they will hunt tirelessly, motivated by hunger, sustained by body fat stores and an occasional grouse or rodent. When the pack kills a large animal they will eat until gorged, relax and digest, then gorge again. It is only during this temporary abundance that daytime rest will occur. The logic is simple and yet perfect. A full belly tells the body to remain quiet and shift into converting food into fat and storing it. That fat will then sustain the wolf as needed in the future. When food is plentiful and kills are frequent, wolves do not become obese. Instead, nature and evolution prescribe that during times of abundance, more wolf pups are born. Wolves are pack animals and there is benefit to the pack as its numbers increase. The elk that is hunted by the wolf is an herbivore, eating primarily grass. Grass as a food source is not a highly packed source of nutrition. Therefore, the elk must graze continually throughout the day and travel to water to get enough to eat. Again, when it fills its belly, the elk will rest as the food is converted into fat. The elk is driven by nature to keep its belly full as the winter snow will all too soon cover the grass and induce a season of deprivation. Elk without a store of fat in the fall will starve to death before the spring rains replenish the grass. Years of abundant spring rain result in more grass growing thicker and more widespread. Less work is required to find its food so the elk can spend more time digesting and forming fat. This results in more calves being born and rapid growth to a size large enough to survive winter. This sedentary behavior of fat formation is optimum activity for elk survival and it is perfectly natural that the elk seek this condition. Needless to say, the factors that effect elk and wolf survival are much more complicated than this simple analysis. What this simple example is designed to show is how fundamental, basic, and perfectly natural it is for humans to seek a state of satiation and sedentary fat conversion.

Humans have spent most of their waking hours for the last 100,000 years, seeking this state. The more time an animal can spend in this state, the more likely it has the biochemical fuel{fat} necessary to reproduce. The more likely it is to pass on its particular genome to its progeny which, sadly to say, is the goal of survival and reproduction. In the quest of modern man to accomplish tremendous feats in science, the arts, engineering, scientific discovery, philosophy, capital accumulation, political power, athletic achievement, or just who catches the biggest damn fish. Stop.

You won't believe this. How successful an individual of a species is dependent on how many grandchildren you have. This is not just arcane environmental ecology theory. If you take the time to study the subject it makes sense. Animals and plants and insects go to tremendous lengths to reproduce, huge self-inflicted expenditures and sacrifices for the result of reproduction. From a perspective of evolutionary ecology, there is not direct benefit from reproduction.

Let's look at a pair of ladybugs as an example. Many if not all of the offspring of a pair of ladybugs will die this year. This means that those two lady bugs put their effort and material into an effort that yielded no benefit to them. It is only when the offspring of the two ladybugs survive long enough to reproduce themselves that the ladybug reproduction is deemed successful. As individuals we do some of this, as parents and grandparents put away money for future college educations, for instance, so a lot of this behavior is "perfectly natural." Part of the reason I point some of this out now is that by the time we get to the end of this book, I'm going to implore you to engage in some "unnatural behavior". What we are going to talk about in terms of food and exercise are going to run contrary to your natural inclinations. The goal is going to be to provide you with the knowledge and disciplines to enjoy a happy, productive, and active life, well into old age. Look around you. That is not the norm. A large fraction of people are already getting fat in their twenties. Most people in their forties and fifties are so physically inept they are incapable of any arduous physical activity. What we are going to teach you in this book and in a series of dvds is going to keep this from happening to you. We are going to keep things relatively simple. There isn't a single breakthrough idea, diet scheme, workout technique, or life-altering epiphany to be found in these pages. What you will find is a lot of common sense, numerous small steps you can reasonably implement, efficiencies you can capture, burdens you can cut out. The goal is feeling good and getting the most enjoyment out of every day that you do have left on this earth. This process of becoming truly physically fit will not only allow you to enjoy all of your activities more fully. It will help eliminate a couple of the worst anxieties people have about aging. Becoming fit will go a long way toward reducing anxiety about what the future holds for your health. You are going to have a much greater feeling of control over that future. As you get stronger, you will feel less threatened by an increasingly younger and faster world. Again, a lot of what we are going to be doing runs contrary to what the natural animal in you wants to do. It is entirely likely that you are already familiar with the tug of war between the donut and the carrot, the sofa and the Stair-master. We're not going to eliminate that struggle, but we'll show you some common sense ways to have both. After all, I like Mexican food and beer as much as I like training, and a very big goal is to be able to **enjoy everything**. There is no guilt in an éclair that is accompanied by a hundred sit-ups. In the process, your abs are stronger, you really enjoyed that pastry and there is no self-loathing. So along the way we'll employ our human intellect to balance out and counter some of our natural tendencies. Nothing new there.

NUTRITION AND WEIGHT CONTROL

Are you overweight? For most people the answer is "yes." If that's the case then it means you have accumulated excess fat over time. Part of becoming truly physically fit is eliminating the excess fat. We're not talking about eliminating all the fat, because maintaining a thin layer of fat under your skin happens to be good for you. By *thin* we mean if you can pinch a half inch to an inch on your butt, thigh and abs you're probably just right. It is also true that a few people are underweight. Most of these folks suffer a shortfall in the amount of muscle they have developed and will benefit from the exercise portions of this program. So tell me, what kind of eater are you? What patterns of eating have resulted in the extra fat? Are you the carnivore who makes a big kill every day and gorges until you are stuffed? Are you the herbivore grazer who nibbles and snacks all day until you don't really know the total amount because you have eaten eighteen mini meals all day? Do you make a habit of eating the wrong kinds of foods most of the time? Not sure? Well, give it some thought. This is not an exercise in guilt identification. You're going to need to identify behavior patterns in the process of planning your changes.

Most people who are overweight have been on some form of a diet in the past, had varying degrees of success in terms of weight loss, and then gained the weight back over time. As you already know, there are a million diet plans out there and what we're going to talk about is **not** another diet plan. There are exotic, absurd, breakthrough and fad diets galore out there. I'm going to tell you right here and now to stay away from all of them. Any diet that tells you to eat copious amounts of fat or no carbohydrates or forty pomegranates a day is a scientifically unproven fad and you are the guinea pig. They will probably work short term, you may well lose weight, but you aren't likely to spend the rest of your life eating like that. There are long established regimented menu programs that will work if you follow them faithfully. You have to ask yourself a couple of questions. Do I or do I not have the discipline to alter what and how I eat? If the answer is no, then one of the plans like Jenny Craig or Weight Watchers just to name two, is a really good way to go. It's simple. It's varied. The only discipline you need is to not cheat on the plan. Stick to the program.

As you read through this book, we will note there are times in life when complication is a necessity. Fundamental analysis of a stock. Flying to the moon. This is not one of them. You can make things complicated and involved but on the subject of fitness such complication is usually a detriment. Remember, we are always looking for simple. By the way, we are also looking for relatively inexpensive options as well. A simple program, a simpler plan. This makes things easier to follow. Less for you to have to figure out. Less likely to get distracted by options and calculations and costs. You will be less likely to let the subconscious mind divert your effort. Simpler is better. We also do not want costs to be a burden or a deterrent. We also insist on sound medical science. These commercially available diet plans are nutritionally complete. Most of them leave you a little hungry part of the time, which is a good thing. Remember back to our discussion of the history of man. Humans evolved under conditions where being a little hungry most of the time was the norm. In modern times, where food is so abundant and affordable in America, even the poorest segments of society are afflicted with epidemic levels of obesity. As far as the human animal is concerned, being able to eat high calorie food every time you feel a twinge of hunger is not normal. It may seem normal to you since that is very likely what you have known your entire life. As far as your body is concerned, it is not normal. And it is definitely not healthy. When you examine the list of diseases that are directly related or exacerbated by obesity, it is very, very long. As we discuss the feeding of the human animal, we don't intend to make you an expert on nutrition or micronutrients or nutriceuticals or phytonutrients or any of the other big words you've heard. We're going to stick to simple common sense. In all likelihood, at this age, you already have a pretty good idea what good nutrition is. So at this point let's say you've decided to pick a well respected, widely known commercial program and stick to it. Good. You're done. Combine that with the exercise we have for you and you'll do well.

Let's say you've looked at yourself and decided you're not a diet plan person. You believe you have the self discipline it takes to decide for yourself what you're going to eat and keep it within reason. That's good too. That's what I do. In that case we're going to provide you with some very simple and common sense eating guidelines to remind yourself of. Most of this you have already heard at some point. **This time you are listening, you are paying attention and you will get it**.

One of the first concepts to get your head around is embracing a little hunger. I don't mean being so desperately hungry that you get all weak and shaky. I mean not satisfying every twinge of hunger by putting food in your mouth. You will learn to recognize that when you are hungry, your body's enzymatic machinery will go to your fat cells and extract the food you need. Now a drawback to hunger is that your body will also try to consume muscle tissue for energy. Since you will be exercising, you'll push that back the other way. But that feeling of a little hunger is your reminder that things are going in the right direction. Now if the hunger gets strong enough, and it will, where some days you just want rid of it, remember, you can eat a piece of fresh fruit or a vegetable or two. Or even three. Until the craving has passed. You need not ever feel desperately hungry. You can, in a moment of compulsive consumption, eat carrots until you are ready to puke and not ingest very many calories. What you don't do is grab a bag of chips. Or slam a cheeseburger. Again, this is mostly common sense. Most of what we will discuss regarding food you already know. Or sort of know. I know that you have heard it before.

Embracing hunger. At first, a completely unpleasant thought. Until you really think about the consequences that lie in store for those who never grasp the concept of embracing hunger. Again, remember, we're not talking about feeling all weak and shaky from starvation, just a little hungry. Now when you're all in tune with the stretching and range of motion program and you're working the muscular strength and endurance components of the program and you're burning calories training, well guess what? Now it's time to eat! So what do I get to eat? The answer is. Everything! Within reason, of course. So let's start talking about what is reasonable. We already know you are going to spend part of most days feeling a little hungry. So let's start talking about the fun part of the day – the eating! You are going to get to eat one **BIG** meal a day. Not two. And not three. So every day that you have to deal with this feeling of hunger, you also get to experience a full belly. This is important on many levels. Psychologically it is important to know that your self imposed deprivation is temporary and will be relieved in a few short hours. Additionally, you are in control of the relief you desire. When you are hungry you know you are doing well and when you eat you are absolved of guilt. Now let's talk about eating, 'cause I like to eat everything. One of the great things about exercising all the time is that you get to eat more. Yes there are limits and you will bump up against them here and there, as eating can result in weight gain or interfere with your workout schedule.

Let's say that you are able and inclined to write your own food schedule. I am. What we're going to talk about in the next segment are some very basics of nutrition, assuming you have common sense and common knowledge of nutrition. There will be a strict adherence to sound medical science, simple and easy to follow formulations, nothing fad or grandiose or Hollywood or South Beach.

I am a firm believer in eating a light breakfast. That does not mean that you have to. If you want to make your BIG meal of the day three eggs, sausage, hash browns with cheese, toast and peaches go ahead. For me, it kind of slows me down. Now, I like doing that once every month or two, just not regularly. Especially at fifty-two, I like to start the day with a bowl of high fiber cereal and a piece of fruit. It's light; it makes it easier to keep going with some proper sustenance in you. Now all of you know the difference between oatmeal and fruit loops. There are a couple of cereals that I like to eat on a regular basis in the morning and you will find yours. What you are looking for is high fiber, low fat, etc. Duh! Whether fruit is included in your cereal or not, you will likely be eating a piece of fruit along with your morning cereal. They just go together. Until you come up with a better plan, figure on fruit and cereal in the morning. It is a real hard combo to beat. Let's say you get used to a light breakfast. That is a really good start.

By the time lunch comes around you are already feeling a little hungry and you are into phase two of your eating strategy. Lunch could be your big meal of the day or it could be another light meal. For me the determining factor is what type of workout I intend for that day and when I'll get to it. We will talk about workout schedules in another segment of this book, but I like to alternate a heavy workout one day and a light workout the next. There is no way I'm doing a heavy workout after a big meal. If it's a light workout day I might make lunch my big meal of the day. In which case I'll eat pretty much whatever I want up to the point of feeling slightly full but not so stuffed that I'm immobilized. That way I can still recover for a light evening workout. If it is a heavy workout day, then I eat something light at lunch. Just enough to take the edge off the hunger. A bowl of beans. A smallish sandwich. A big melon.

I get my major workout in from four to six-thirty. Then I'll eat my big meal that night. By now you are getting the idea. This is, of course, not rocket science. Primarily common sense. I heard a fellow say some years ago, "I used to live to eat, now I eat to live". That is not a bad philosophy. However, I like to shoot for something in the middle. I seldom let my eating or drinking get in the way of my activity schedule. On the other hand, my activity schedule allows me to enjoy eating all kinds of yummy food and drinking beer. We are going to go over a few fundamentals of nutrition next.

Back to our original question. Are you too fat? If you are, then you will suffer a period of relative deprivation until your enhanced workout schedule burns off the fat and you can get to your steady state where your activity level is burning off your consumptive level. So let's say you have achieved your desired weight and you have your workout schedule going. At this point it is important to realize that you now get to vary things up a bit, going up and down five pounds is not a problem. You can take a cruise on a ship and go a little over the top on the eating at those gorgeous spreads of food or have a lazy weekend of pampering at the spa or fishing or whatever without working out. A big part of getting down to a desirable weight is it gives you a little wiggle room as to variety in your regimen. If you get off track a little enjoying life's pleasures and indulgences, you are not far off course. Let's talk a little bit about some basic fundamentals of nutrition. Again, we're going to stick to common sense, simplicity and good science.

You need protein for muscle repair and development as well as enzymatic functions. You only need about four ounces of protein a day. That's not much. Anything above and beyond that gets burned for energy or converted to fat and stored. You need carbohydrates for energy. It is basic fuel. Complex carbohydrates like starches are better than simple carbohydrates like sugars. You need a little bit of fat as there are biochemical processes that are dependent on certain minimal amounts of the right kinds of fats. Most of the fat we eat gets stored as fuel so getting essential fatty acids is pretty easy. If you are eating quality, healthy food, it's in there. I take a daily dose of fish oil to make certain I get my omega-3's. I make sure it is metal free. There is ample evidence that these valuable oils assist heart, brain, and joint function. You can get them from flax seed oil if you are concerned about a little fishy aftertaste. You need fiber. Fiber is the bulk volume that pushes all the crap through your system and keeps you regular. If you are sticking to a diet of a wide variety of whole grains, fruits, vegetables, seeds, and nuts, you are going to be getting a lot of fiber. Finally, you need myriad vitamins and coenzymes and minerals that are present in all types of healthy foods. If you are eating good food, you will probably get enough of all of them. If you want to be certain, you can take a multivitamin supplement. I do. Most of those vitamins go right through you and down the drain. That's fine. They're cheap and I'm confident I'm getting all my vitamins and minerals and I don't have to calculate anything. I also add a dose of glucosamine and chondroitin for my joints.

So let's get back to what you are going to be eating most of the time and we'll build sort of a food pyramid. You can't beat seeds. Seeds are almost perfect little packages of food. Many foods made from seeds suffer from being processed, so we'll keep our eye on that as we look at food. Beans are seeds. Beans are an incredible little package of complex carbohydrates, proteins, vitamins, and minerals. You just can't beat them. Whole grain breads are made from ground up seeds of wheat and oats and rye. Good stuff. It is the whole grain part that is very important. There are a lot of very yummy bread choices out there that have some portion of the nutritive value removed. Portuguese sweet bread, croissants, tortillas. I'm not saying they are bad for you. Just try to stick to that whole grain label as much as possible.

Nuts are seeds. Same idea. Now, nuts have a little more fat in them than grains so you will keep that in mind as you dive into a can. Still they are full of lots of good stuff. This brings us back to the concept that one type of seed is rich in this micronutrient and another is rich in that so if you are eating different and varied seeds you get a wide variety of micronutrients. Remember the old P&J sandwich? Make it with whole grain bread and real fruit preserves and you got yourself one fine sandwich my friend! You already know that fruit is good for you. Fruit is the package that the plant produced to induce animals to consume and spread the seed of the plant. Now the seed may or may not be an edible part of the fruit. You will eat the peach but not the pit. You eat a banana, seeds and all. As you already know, the fruit has just enough of the natural sugar fructose to make it taste sweet enough to eat. Which is good for you of course because you get a bunch of fiber and a few micronutrients as well as a low calorie filler all in one package. And when you eat a piece of fruit the best thing of all is that

YOU DID NOT EAT A DONUT! Don't get me wrong, I like donuts too. It's just that at fifty- two I get a lot more bananas than éclairs.

Vegetables are a very similar story with less fructose and more vitamins. So as part of your nutritional plan, you are going to try to include as many veggies as will fit. Having a ham sandwich? Pile it to the ceiling with tomato and lettuce. Try replacing the mayo with applesauce, it tastes great. Of course you started with whole grain bread. Most of your bean and soup recipes will have a lot of veggies in them. You can find a plethora of canned or dried soup and bean products in your local supermarket. You will find a lot of really good – and cheap - stuff there. Keep an eye on the sodium content. Some of them will be relatively high in sodium and you might steer away from them. It is not hard to read from the daily allowances label on the back. If you suffer from hypertension your doctor will have advised you to play close attention to your sodium intake. Another advantage to your increased workout schedule is that you can eat a little more sodium as you will be sweating it out. My blood pressure is 120/80 so I don't worry about salt very much. In fact I put salt on my tomatoes and melons.

Now, what about dessert? Well, dessert is dessert. Yummy, fun, nutritionally void empty calories probably full of bad cholesterol prone to predisposing humans to obesity and disease and rolls of ugly fat, did I mention yummy and fun? You will decide how much of that pleasure fits into your plan. The same goes for alcohol. Although doctors do assign a few more beneficial attributes to wine and beer than dessert, they are in a similar boat in that they are rewards and pleasures you get to enjoy as a result of your hard work and should be enjoyed in relatively small quantities with absolutely no guilt.

It is worthy of repeating the magnitude and varying ways exercise helps your health. My cholesterol and triglyceride level just recently got on to the scale. I've been below the scale for many years now. Let me say a couple of more things about the science of nutrition. There are some very good sources of genuinely useful knowledge about nutrition. A couple of examples are the You docs, Mehmet Oz and Michael Roizen, both medical doctors. Another excellent source is Andrew Weil, MD. These men have scoured the research, actively practiced their art and science and written several outstanding books that you can dive into and learn a great deal of specifics about the myriad biochemicals that make up the science of nutrition. If you are the type of person who wishes to learn the details of what you should and should not be eating, these gents are very good sources.

I have studied enough biochemistry to know that when it comes to food, I just don't want to try that hard. Since my training helps keep my lab values in good shape, I don't have to scrutinize every morsel that crosses my lips. I like to stick to a simple common sense approach. I know (as do you) what is healthy food and what is junk food. So I eat healthy food most of the time and I enjoy a little junk food occasionally. Just to say I did, I'm going to give you two lists. The first list is a bunch of good words to find on your food packages and nutriceutical supplement labels: HDL, anti-oxidant, anti-inflammatory, turmeric, lycopene, lutein, tocopherols, Co-Q-10, flavonoids, proanthocyanids, alpha-lipoic acid, ginger, DHEA, artic root, reishi, ginseng, ginkgo biloba, astragalus, silymarin, carotenoids, anthrocyanins, omega-3, polyphenols, grass fed meat, extra virgin olive oil, glucosamine, and chondroitin. The list of bad words you want to minimize in your food are trans fat, artificial, LDL, triglycerides, omega-6, partially hydrogenated, grain fed meat, and shortening. So there you are. With all the information there is to glean from this book we've spent maybe five pages on nutrition. It is not because it lacks importance. It is just that it need not be complicated.

You can buy a hundred diet books and spend a thousand hours and confuse yourself into a convoluted knot about nutrition and you will be no farther along than if you follow the basic simple principles outlined here. In all likelihood you would be worse off if you start down the path on some idiot diet plan that compels you to eat all fat or no carbohydrates or some other unsustainable baloney. By this age you know that diets do not work. You may well lose weight, but it does not last. The only unnatural concept you need to embrace and apply your intellect to is the value of self-imposed hunger. Again, there is nothing that bad about mild and temporary periods of hunger. You are going to get really good at that in a short amount of time, similarly to any other strategy you have learned. You are in control, it is not fanatically regimented, and if you miss a few days you just get back on the wagon. Now if I intended to sell you on some complicated and involved program that required that you stick to some regimented schedule of ingesting 86 grams of this and 250mgs of that every fourteen hours and required that you get away from the fundamental precepts of food I could probably write another fifty pages on the subject. But there is no need for that. Most of what you need to do you already know. Some of what you need to change you already know.

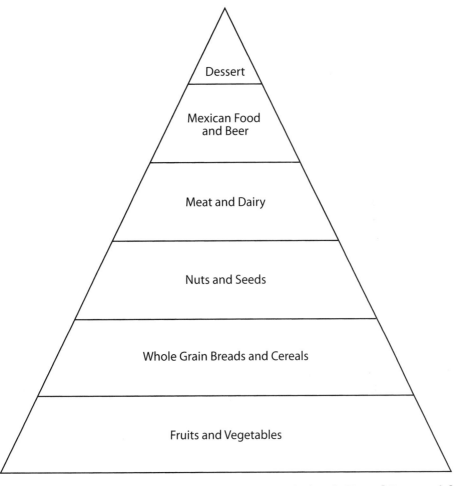

Brian's Food Pyramid

FLEXIBILITY AND RANGE OF MOTION

In the process of developing and maintaining your highest physical condition, you may not have become aware of the need and value of flexibility and range of motion exercises. Most people get to a very advanced age and never learn about the value of maintaining flexibility and range of motion. Most people never feel the need to do so, or fail to realize how much such exercises can benefit their health. Sure, everyone knows you're supposed to stretch, even though hardly anyone does. This is really sad, as a great deal of seniors' health problems could be reduced if they learned to do these exercises. I am amazed at the number of high level athletes who do not grasp these concepts. I train with advanced belt martial artists and professional athletes who are virtually ignorant of flexibility and range of motion exercises. These are younger athletes. Most of them are getting by on youth and natural ability, never recognizing or achieving their maximum potential, in part because they fail to see the value in this type of training.

I was close to fifty years old before a significant portion of this aspect of training became relevant to me. I had trained in the martial arts as a young man. Like most, when I was young, I got by on natural flexibility. In the years between twenty and fifty, I failed to learn the value of flexibility and range of motion training. Like many of you, in the years between my youth and my present age, I just lived my life. It was an active life that included many forms of exercise, with no disciplined or regimented workout schedule. I rode my bike, hunted, chopped wood, and chased my kids around. All that stuff is good. Unfortunately, if you want to be truly physically fit and are capable into your fifties and beyond you will need to follow a complete fitness plan that encompasses all aspects of fitness. The good news is you have found it! The bad news is, you have to do it. Well not really bad news. A sobering realization? Not quite an epiphany. Maybe just facing reality. Anyway, that is what you are here for. We are going to teach you how to do the types of exercises that are going to make you look better, feel better and enjoy the remaining years of your life to the fullest possible potential. In the process, you are going to have more and better sex. You are going to enjoy more of a feeling of control over your life. And you are going to have less fear about what the future holds for you. As you improve your ability to move yourself about and improve your health at the same time, some of the anxiety that we all have regarding what is in store for you will lessen. You will know that you are making a serious and yet reasonable effort to insure your health and your mobility well into old age. At the same time you won't have to become fanatical about any aspect of this plan.

As the years have gone by, you have probably done a little of this and a little of that in terms of getting exercise. That is perfectly normal. Most of us have so many economic and familial obligations that the concept of staying in shape gets relegated to the back burner. Exercise is something we know we should do but has a hard time rising high enough on the priority list to actually get to it.

When most folks are in their twenties and early thirties, they can get by on youthful vigor and keep up quite a busy pace without a specific exercise plan. Most can carry an extra twenty pounds of fat as well. Somewhere in the mid-thirties these behaviors begin to catch up with you. By the time you get to forty, if you are carrying extra weight and not actively exercising, your ass is draggin'. You're tired, lack energy and your feet and joints and back are starting to really hurt. It is unfortunate that at this point most people give in to the increased difficulty of moving around and things proceed downhill from there. If a person can't get motivated to turn their ship in a better direction, it becomes increasingly difficult to reverse a pattern of sedentary behavior as time goes by. That is why the time to start is, as it always is, now.

You have no doubt heard enough reports of the obesity epidemic in this country. Most people who are overweight have the idea that they are "a little heavy". Most are in denial of the magnitude of the negative affect of being overweight or obese has on their health. Most plan to lose the extra weight and start exercising "real soon.".If everyone who is relatively young and overweight knew of the large number of diseases that are exacerbated by excess fat, knew of the diseases they were predisposing themselves to, and knew how much easier it is to turn their ship at an earlier age, we would all be better off. The health care costs of treating obesity-related disease are staggering. Remember this. This is the first generation in which obesity is affecting a significant number of children. In the entire realm of human existence, this is the first time there were significant numbers of fat children. The financial burden imposed on society as this generation ages through the medical system will be staggering. These children do not know any better. Their ability to choose what to eat is no better than their ability to choose what to watch on TV. If they have overweight or obese parents offering an example of sedentary behavior, then this pattern is likely to be engrained in them. Anyone who is capable of doing a rational and realistic assessment of themselves and their kids, and comes to the conclusion that changes must be made, is now at least looking in the right direction.

So now you are looking in the right direction. I kid you not, this is the first step down a new path to a healthier and happier you. I could toss in a bunch of tired old clichés right here and they would actually fit! And they would actually be true. A lifelong journey begins with the first step. You only fail when you quit. Two steps up, one step back. You can lead a horse to water. Does a bear poop in the woods? Oops, sorry.........

One of the best and relatively easy aspects of an exercise program that I like to see people start with involves flexibility and range of motion. It is absolutely vital to the success of any fitness plan that a person spend a balanced amount of time and effort on each area of that plan. Flexibility and range of motion training will go a long way to helping ensure you do not sustain an injury that sets you back. It also will do more to reduce your level of pain from either strong exercise or sedentary behavior than anything else you do. Remember, a diet is not likely to succeed long term without exercise.

Flexibility and range of motion exercises are fundamental to all other forms of fitness training. Usually you will want to do these types of exercises prior to your muscular strength and endurance exercises. When your time is limited (and whose isn't?), these become the most important aspect of fitness. They are also easier to fit into small increments throughout the day without working up a sweat. Invariably you will feel better after you do them. Anyone who has received any training in yoga or tai chi will understand this, because there is a lot of overlap in the motions. When we talk about flexibility and range of motion, we are talking about your body's ability to move.

When you were around sixteen or seventeen years old, you had your greatest degree of natural flexibility and range of motion. You could stretch as far as you were genetically designed to and your joints allowed the maximum amount of movement. From then on, two things began to happen. You began to thicken. It started with increased muscle mass as a part of maturation. Perhaps you took on a physically demanding job or sporting activity that built muscle. Next, you probably began to lay down a layer of fat (some people did this more than others). You may have taken on work that was primarily sedentary. As time marched on, unless you studied yoga or tai chi, you lost range of motion and flexibility.

Let's examine flexibility. Flexibility primarily refers to your muscles and tendons, your ability to stretch. Most of you have a pretty good idea what muscles are and what they do. We're going to elaborate a little bit. You can feel your arm or leg as you contract a muscle and tell approximately where that muscle is. If you're lucky it gets hard. Your muscles' job is to contract. That means they get shorter when they are performing their function. That function is designed to move you or something else to do useful work. Muscles have no inherent ability to elongate. You need to apply your generous brain capacity to an opposing set of muscles to elongate and stretch a particular muscle that you want to get longer. Muscle tissue does not like to be stretched. Initially when you stretch a muscle, it will try to contract to "fight" the stretch and you will gently and firmly hold your stretches for twenty to thirty seconds to overcome this normal phenomenon. More on technique later, we're still talking theory.

A big part of stretching muscle tissue involves time. I'm going to make a point here and I'm going to remind you of it so often you will get tired of reading it and hearing it. By then it will be seared into your brain like one of those little ditties that plays over and over in your head and you will be able to remind yourself for the two or three years it will take to get your body back into tip-top working order. It has taken a long time for you to lose range of motion and flexibility. It will take a couple of years to get it back. If you stick with this, you will get it back, at least most of it. And since this is likely your last go-around (I would love to believe in reincarnation but I just don't have anything solid to go on), look down the road. Say you are fifty. Statistics give you approximately thirty more years. Do you want to sit on the couch, stiff, and in pain? Weak and fearful? Sickly and sexually frustrated? Dismissed as old, frail and incapable? Hell no you don't. I know that a couple of years may seem like forever in a society where instant gratification is the norm. But those years will pass by anyway and the question is "How good are you going to feel then?" Well, you have seen hundreds of diets and hundreds of workouts come and go. Most of them promise dramatic results with little effort and they all fail.

Back to the subject of stretching muscle tissue. Muscle tissue is in a constant state of being rebuilt. When you continually and regularly contract muscle[when you work out a lot] muscle rebuilds thicker and stronger. Individual subunits of muscle tissue are replaced and added to and a muscle gets bigger. During this continuous process, if you continually stretch, the muscle it will be rebuilt at a minutely longer length than it was before. And I do mean minutely. If you try to elongate a muscle rapidly you will tear it. This, quite obviously, is an injury that you do not want. This can set your progress back weeks to months. In the process of being diligent and persistent at progress we will be equally careful that we do not overdo it. So when it comes to muscle tissue, slow and steady progress is the goal. This way the muscle gets thicker and stronger and longer over time. We'll teach you a bunch of specific techniques on that later on. Right now we are talking about theory and goals. The end result you hope to obtain is lean, hard and flexible muscle tissue with no tears. Now muscles are able to affect useful work by exerting the force of contraction on a bone. The bone is the lever that actually does something like throw a ball or scratch your hiney. The muscle is attached to the bone by the tendon, and the tendon is a very important part of this scenario.

The tendon is made of dense fibrous tissue that is very difficult if not impossible to stretch. It is very tough. Tendons can be stretched over time and lucky for you, the effort you make to stretch your muscle will stretch your tendon at the same time. The tendon is like a rope, made of multiple small strands, woven together into a tough fibrous connection that neither shortens nor elongates under normal use. The way you can stretch a tendon is this. As with almost all tissue, individual sub-units of that tissue are being replaced over time. As wear and tear occurs, individual strands are replaced. How fast this happens is called the "turnover rate.' For the collagenous tissue that makes up a tendon, the turnover rate is about one year. In other words, it takes about one year to replace any given tendon. So you can see how this is a time-consuming process. Your body's mechanism for tendon renewal is inserting one new strand at a time, and if you are stretching, each new one is minutely longer than the one it replaced. You can build up your muscle mass and strength in a few months if you really go at it, but stretching of muscle and tendon take time. That is fine. You are going to be at this for the rest of your life, so that you can move and enjoy and shimmy and shake, strut your stuff and eat your cake.

You now have a thumbnail sketch of flexibility. You are used to thinking of it as how far you can stretch, which is a very good approach. Flexibility,range of motion, and stretching are overlapping and interrelated concepts. One most certainly affects the other. Range of motion describes how well your joints are able to move. The attendant muscles and tendons will also limit joint movement to some extent. Certain joints such as your knee move front to back in one direction with very little lateral deviation and that's it. There is little you are going to improve in terms of range of motion involving a knee. Maybe I spoke to soon. If you injure a knee and can't bend it and have to go through physical therapy to get that ability back, yes, you can improve range of motion in a knee. What we are talking about is going to be your joints that move in several directions (or at least joints that used to). Your hips and shoulders and neck and spine. Your ankles and wrists and elbows. These are joints that you will be spending a fair amount of time on for the remainder of your life, maintaining and improving their range of motion.

Your joints are made up of connections between two bones. By this I mean two articulating or movable bones. Those two bones are attached primarily by ligaments. Ligaments have a lot of properties similar to tendons. They are made up of tough collagenous tissue that is not easily stretched. When they are torn, they take a long time to heal. Pain in a ligament, which means pain in a joint, is something we are very attentive to. We do not ignore pain in a joint. You heard the DI bark "No pain, no gain!" That does not apply to ligaments. This is a good time to bring up a point that I will repeat (remember, repetition is learning). If you ever have pain in a joint when you are stretching, stop. Reexamine the stretch for proper technique and do something else if need be. Ligaments are tissue that will get stretched a little, inadvertently as your muscle and tendon stretches. During your range of motion exercises you will be impeded and limited to some extent by the ligaments. Truth is, it may be impossible to tell which type of tissue is limiting your motion without the aid of biometric analysis. In most cases you do not need to know. Just remember the rule about pain in a joint. If you have pain in a joint when stretching, stop.

This brings up another little aside. You are completely aware of the "little aches and pains" you experience. Most of these you shrug off and keep going, while some hurt enough to limit your activity. In the process of performing these exercises you will feel little aches and pains on a regular basis. Only you can tell if it is a large enough pain to feel like an impending injury. Only you can make that call. When something hurts enough to persuade you to back off, do not despair for there are so many exercises to do that you could not possibly get to all of them in a day anyway. So you will simply do something else. As I will tell you again, there are days when my elbow tells me, "You're not doing pushups today," for no apparent reason. So I do something else, probably more leg lifts. Remember that if something hurts, you need not avoid activity altogether. The one possible exception to this is back pain. Sometimes my back hurts enough that I can do nothing. We'll talk about that more in another section.

Back to range of motion. You will see various range of motion exercises in this book and the supplemental videos that will show you how to get your shoulders, hips, neck, back, and ankles to return to the full range of motion you had when you were much younger. Keep in mind that the series of exercises you see take me about thirty-five minutes a day and I do them every day. On a good day, I get to do them twice. I will do them prior to every big workout. Ideally that is every other day. On the light workout days, I do range of motion and flexibility exercises and stick work, the filipino martial art of arnis. Some days it seems I do not have time for anything, as I do not always get to make my schedule fit my workouts. As often as not, I have to make my workouts fit my schedule. This is something almost all of you will have to deal with at some time or another. One really helpful aspect to this part of your training is that you can get it in bits and pieces throughout your day. If you can't devote thirty-five minutes to it at one time there is a really good chance that you can find five minutes here and three minutes there throughout your day that add up quickly. As I said before, don't worry about looking silly swinging your arms around. Anyone who is aware of what you are trying to accomplish will think it's cool. Most of those who think it is weird are probably in a state of physical condition that could benefit from the same activity. Most of them probably feel weak and tired, the very feelings you are working to overcome. So what the hell do you care what they think anyway? At some point in the future they will come across this information and they will look back and remember Mary in shipping working her shoulder and realize how enlightened that activity was. Shortly you will get into the pages that demonstrate these flexibility and range of motion exercises. I promised you this book would be short and sweet, with no filler. I am a simple man. This is a simple plan.

MUSCULAR STRENGTH AND ENDURANCE

Muscles. This is the part of being in shape that is intuitive to all. Ask a little kid about who is strong and in shape and he will point to a picture of a bodybuilder. Fortunately we are a little smarter than most little kids and realize that being in the kind of physical condition a bodybuilder has developed is not our goal. Strong muscles are good. Well defined muscles are good. Big muscles are not so good. Let me amend that. If you are in your twenties and you are looking to show off to attract the opposite sex, big muscles are about as useful as breast implants. They turn heads, might help you get laid, and they can enhance your self esteem, but in the long run will fail you. If you are much over forty, the idea of building big muscles and having six pack abs is a counterproductive one. By now you have outgrown some of your adolescent delusions.

At some point guys realize that breast implants just aren't real. Gals realize that big biceps do not translate into responsibility, productivity, reliability, humor, and kindness, the qualities that will sustain a relationship over time or enhance good parenting skills. So now that we are forty- to fifty-something, let's get to the reality of what the concepts of muscular strength and endurance can do to make our lives better. It was only a few short years ago that I used to spend a majority of my weekends working on my domicile. Carpentry, plumbing, planting, concrete, fencing, you name it. I actually did not mind it most of the time. I liked getting things done, saved some money. I was happy to know it was done right. But it hurt. It was activity and certainly it was exercise, but it was not good quality exercise. And it hurt. All over. At fifty-two I am glad that I'm almost done and I genuinely go out of my way to avoid home improvement and repair projects.

This concept is kind of important. Most of you gals out there probably, statistically, don't do a lot of home improvement and repair work. I know my wife doesn't. You guys probably do. To be able to have the time to train and develop your fitness and health, you are both going to have to try to avoid wanting, asking for, and doing home improvement projects, unless you have the ability to pay someone else to do them. I have heard people advocate yard work and gardening as a form of exercise and I'm not so arrogant as to call them foolish or wrong. It is just that it has been in my experience that those kinds of activities (and you can add roofing and plastering in as well), do not result in the quality exercise that you will get when you engage in the techniques shown in this book.

At or about the age of fifty, the kind of muscle you want to develop is lean and hard. You do not want big muscles. There are several reasons why, and we will get into them shortly. The kind of muscle you want to develop is the kind you can maintain and utilize for useful function for the rest of your life. This type is going to have the added benefit of strengthening your joints at the same time, and give you a dose of endurance [cardio] work as well. Most of the home improvement and yard work type of exercise is not good for your joints or your back. You seldom stretch sufficiently, seldom warm up, and often go from a resting state to lifting something heavy in short order. None of that is good. I know doing home improvement projects is good for your house and sense of pride and accomplishment. I have done a million of them over the years, but it is not good for your health. What you will be doing in the muscular strength portion of your training regimen is using relatively light weights, from five to thirty pounds, lifting your own body parts, legs and torso, and doing a lot of repetitions. This will do several things for you at the same time. It will develop good muscular strength for the specific muscles you are working. If done at a relatively rapid pace, it will provide a portion of your endurance or heart muscle work at the same time. You will work on your balance. And it will save you time. If you are like most folks, you will have a hard time finding enough time for all of this. We are going to show you ways to be more efficient in your workouts, allowing you to accomplish more in a given amount of time.

Muscular strength is important on several levels. Naturally, when you were young, you took strength for granted. Some people had more than others, and chances are you had enough to suit your needs or you did what it took to develop more. Now that you are fifty, you realize that you have about one-half the strength you had at twenty. As my four-year-old says, "Oh, well." At this age you want and need to focus on the kind of strength and the amount of strength you need to move you around. Moving you around is the highest priority. Where you want to go, and when you want to go. Minimal limitations. Minimal restrictions. Minimal help. Maximum mobility. And move quickly.

So let's push a little metal and lift a little flesh and get there. There will be several ancillary benefits to this effort as well. You are going to look better as a result of your effort. The value of this is not to be overlooked. You will be more attractive to your sexual partner. This will of course enhance your desirability. This is good. This will enhance your self esteem. Bingo. This is one of those win- win situations that are all too infrequent in life. As you perform the muscular strength exercises in this program, we will try to remind you to perform them at a relatively rapid rate. You will gain two significant benefits from this. Remember we are talking about relatively light weights or your own body weight. If you can lift briskly, you save time. I assume your time to work out is hard to come by. It is for me. I'm one of those nitwits who needed two tries to get the marriage thing right and still have small children at home. You will get more work done in the available time. Second, if you lift quickly, you will add an endurance component to your strength training. Rapid lifting of light weights will get your heart rate up. You will get your breathing rate up. This is your endurance component. You already know that if you jog or ride a bike at a brisk pace you will start breathing faster to keep up. This is good. How fast you need to breathe is a good measure of how hard your heart is working. During your muscular strength training, if you can lift at a faster pace and get your breathing rate up, then you are getting some cardio[heart] work in at the same time. Endurance training is cardiovascular heart muscle training. Endurance training is also training your major muscle groups in your legs and chest and arms to be able to work for a long time. Most of all, endurance training is exercising your heart into a strong enough state to be able to carry you through a long workout, a long walk, a long bike ride or swim, a long life.

Much of the weakening of your muscles that happens as you age is a natural process that cannot be stopped. That being said, you can absolutely reduce the rate at which that weakening occurs. And this is a really cool thing. You can absolutely turn back the clock on this aspect of aging. There are very few areas of the aging process in which you can literally and genuinely turn back the clock. This is one of them. I am not bragging when I tell you that I am in better physical condition than most of the thirty-year-olds you will see. It is not that I am some sort of special individual or uniquely gifted athlete. I exercise a lot, enjoy doing it, eat a healthy diet, and make love to my beautiful forty-year-old wife as often as possible.

As you go through the various lifting exercises in this book, and work on developing your muscular strength and endurance, there are two questions to ask yourself: to How much weight am I going to lift? (and) How many times am I going to lift it? The good news here is that there aren't a lot of rules in this area. You may also vary things around according to how you feel on a given day. A lot of this you probably already know, but we'll go over it again anyway. The number of times you perform a specific lift, say a bicep curl with a twenty pound barbell, is called a repetition. You may do ten, twenty or fifty. Those fifty repetitions constitute one set, as in one set of repetitions. I know this runs counter to what most trainers will tell you, but if I can't do at least twenty reps of some lift in a set then I go to a lighter weight. A lot of trainers have a target number of ten to twelve reps a set. For me, the strain of lifting a weight so heavy that I can only get it up ten times before I am out of gas is just too much. My guess is that those fitness trainers are used to training younger people who are interested in more power. I'm not sure. What I do know is that I have heard and read about that ten to twelve rep strategy over and over throughout the years. I know how it feels and I do not like it. When I am doing my various leg lifting exercises to facilitate my kicks, my goal is one hundred reps.

Remember also that the more the weight, the more the strain on the joints. We want to strengthen the components of your joints by making them perform a lot of a sustainable workload, not an overload. Another aspect of the "less weight-more rep" philosophy is that it is easier to generate an endurance or cardiovascular component to your workout in the same amount of time. And we are always looking for time efficiency. One other aspect of the "lighter weight-more reps-more sets of reps" philosophy is that on any given day I may have one part of my anatomy that informs me that I am not doing push-ups that day. Perhaps my elbow has announced that push-ups are out. So I may do one hundred more squats instead. I know what you are thinking. He said this already. I have heard this before. I repeat myself primarily because you may well need to remind yourself when your elbow hurts that you can still do squats. There will also be days when all of a sudden, instead of doing thirty-five lateral lifts, I feel like doing sixty. When you have a lighter weight you can adapt more easily. You know how at this age there are some days it hurts to get out of bed and you think to yourself, "I didn't do anything yesterday?" Other days you can go and go and you have to use your wisdom to temper your activity so that you don't hurt tomorrow. So as you study the various lifts we will show you, keep in mind that you will not do all of them in any given workout. Some you may not ever do at all. Some you will like more than others and you will have the opportunity to vary them so that you don't get bored.

Now it is a fact that all of these lifts are designed to aid my ability to function as a martial artist. Each and every one of them has some direct application to my conditioning program to allow me to block a strike or throw a kick or move laterally. That being said, I never get bored doing the same lifts over and over because when I can perform some specific martial art move, I know how I developed and maintained the capability. In this tome, I am going to try to convince you of the value of martial arts training as a wonderful form of fitness and confidence enhancement for the remainder of your life. Even if this type of training never appeals to you, and you have some other sport or athletic endeavor you like to engage in, the fundamentals of this program will help you.

In terms of maintaining your health and vigor, it really doesn't matter what recreation or sport you engage in. As a matter of fact, the concept of cross-training is a very good one. Let's assume you have one primary activity you enjoy and would like to enjoy at a relatively high level. Doing some other physical activity here and there to get some different exercise, to use a different set of muscles, is a really good idea. Let's say your preferred form of physical activity is ballroom dancing. The whirl and twirl, the form and grace, music and charm are your cat's meow. That is great. It just so happens that the squats, ankle lifts, and lateral motion exercises you find in this program (those I use for martial arts) will really enable you as a ballroom dancer. I really like to ride a bicycle, and my kids demand I swim all the time. As a result I get something resembling cross-training in the process. I like to spend about one month out of the year hunting in the Rocky Mountains. We go after elk, mule deer, whitetail deer, and antelope. It is great exercise. It is a spiritual reengaging of a primal instinct that was required of males of the human species not more than four or five generations ago. It has been required of males of the human species for more than 100,000years. Not so many years ago, as a male of the human species, if you were not adept at hunting, there was a very good chance that your mate and children would go hungry. If that pattern of behavior persisted, you would not reproduce. As a result, men hunted hard. There were very few social safety nets to help out when one family was experiencing a shortfall of necessities. Obviously in today's society, hunting is not required to obtain meat. You can pay someone else to kill it for you and place it in a plastic wrapped Styrofoam tray at the supermarket for your convenience. Do not get me wrong. There is nothing wrong with paying for a tri tip at the market. I do it. One advantage to harvesting your own meat from the forests of the Rocky Mountains and the prairies of the Great Plains is that you are getting primarily grass fed meat. When you buy primarily grain fed meat, which a lot of beef is, you get a higher ratio of omega-6's compared to an animal that is primarily grass fed. It will be naturally higher in omega-3's. I am not going to try to convince you to take up big game hunting as a recreational activity. The point is that that any physical activity has its merits.

TIME MANAGEMENT

I know what is going through your mind right now. How the hell am I going to find thirty minutes a day to do range of motion and flexibility and another thirty to ninety minutes to do muscular strength and endurance exercises? On the one hand, free time can be really hard to come by. On the other hand, it is easy to waste. If you are a normal human being, and I presume you are, you have more free time in your day being wasted than you realize. Much of it is in the form of two minutes here and four minutes there, dissipated in some mindless activity.

Even in an environment such as the dojo or gym, where people presumably go to workout, I see people standing around chitchatting for ten minutes here and ten minutes there when they could be training. The same thing happens to you at work. Someone comes up to you and starts talking about some subject and before you know it you have spent five minutes in some completely unproductive and likely uninteresting banter. Well, guess what. You did not make any money in that five minutes. And you did not stretch your thighs. Or your shoulders. Or any of the other self-beneficial acts that you are trying to fit into your schedule. If you really take a close look at your schedule tomorrow, you will likely find several periods - anywhere from two to twenty minutes long - that are very poorly spent. In a sense, that is unproductive time. This does not mean that every waking minute must be engaged in productive activity. It should not. There needs to be quiet time to think and reflect and be idle. But you do not want to waste your time listening to some idiot talk about themselves. If you are going to watch some relatively mindless program on TV for entertainment, set it up ahead of time up so you can be working on your flexibility or strength program at the same time. You could call it "multitasking" if you want to sound hip. It only takes a minute to make enough room in front of the TV to stretch.

As you remember from the Flexibility and Range of Motion sections, you can do some of this and some of that any time during the day and it is good to do all of it twice. Let me make a real easy guess. You have a job. And a house. With a mortgage. And maintenance. And kids. And aging parents. And God knows what else you are responsible for. And everybody and their damn brother is dependent on you to be responsible for taking care of their stuff because they are either unable or unwilling to do so. If your immediate family needs your time and effort you are likely to provide it. With children and the elderly, it never ceases. And that is part of the joy and burden of life that we all get to balance. Obviously you are not going to tell your kids to go sit it the corner while you exercise. If your aging parent needs your time, your workout may get interrupted. The times we need to look at are situations such as this one: the kids are at the park for thirty minutes playing on the playground equipment and you are watching them. Do you stretch during that time? Do you do sit-ups? Do you talk to some unintelligent person? Do you care what someone else thinks of you as you go through your range of motion regimen? The answers are(or should be) yes, yes, and no, no. Most of the people who would waste your time talking about what they think are out of shape, overweight, and not all that bright. All of the conditions you are seeking to avoid. Of course you don't want to be rude, but you just don't have the time. It has been my observation in life that most people who seem to have free time in the period of adulthood are either relatively unmotivated and don't have high expectations and therefore not likely to accomplish much. They are willing to accept the very limited gains their efforts will achieve; or they came from money and expect to get stuff anyway. Either way, whoever you are, you do not get to be in good physical condition much past your mid-twenties if you don't work at it. And work takes time, which you must find, or perhaps I should say, make. As you begin to examine your schedule for ways to make time to work out, you may have to look for things that you will cease doing.

As this process moves forward you will be bombarded continually by hundreds of messages about all the things you should be doing. You should buy more life insurance. You should volunteer. You should build a deck, go fishing, go to church, get a sports car, do this, do that, until you realize that you cannot possibly do everything everyone is telling you to do. Many of the things people are imploring you to do will somehow or other involve you putting money in their pocket. Will you get good value for your buck, that buck you must spend time earning and probably paying tax on in order to spend on that sports car? You must decide that. Even this book and video series, in which I will try to convince you of the tremendous value and good result you will achieve, will cost you money. You might spend a little over a hundred dollars on this series and it will return thousands of hours of good health. I can say with absolutely no fear of contradiction that the dollars and time spent exercising will return more to you than almost any other spent.

A few things that will happen as your training progresses. At the very outset you may notice a feeling of being wiped out by an increased workout schedule. That won't last. After a month or so you will notice you have more energy. All day. Even after a workout. It is amazing how much better you will feel. You are going to realize an increase in your productivity at work. Over time the increase in productivity will translate into more dollars earned in a shorter time. It always does. This is one of the truly elegant parts of this equation. The time you spend exercising ends up paying for itself! Think of this point. It does not matter what the field or what the job, someone who is in better physical condition or is better looking has an advantage. People would rather talk to you if you are fit and pretty than fat and ugly. You are more likely to make a sale if you are in shape. Further more, the time spent exercising is not taxed. Many of the activities that you engage in require you spend money. The government has not yet figured out a way to tax you on your sit-ups. That's more important than just a joke. A lot of the things that you are going to spend a great many hours of your life trying to accomplish and have [which means pay for] are going to be subject to taxation.. In other words, they end up costing twenty to fifty percent more than the sticker because the dollars you spend on them are subject to income tax. This concept is important to keep in mind as you weigh your priorities. I am not saying that you should not go skiing or join a tennis club because those are taxable dollars. What I am saying is you should think twice about getting a bigger house or a fancier car or more jewelry. Think in terms of what it costs in dollars, taxable dollars and time. Time spent earning the dollars. Time that you might rather spend on the health benefits of exercise. Don't get me wrong, I recognize that a corvette is going to make you feel good. A corvette would make me feel good, too. It's just that by the time you spend $50K on the car, you spend $25K in interest and $25K in taxes. That corvette cost you $100,000s! Let's say you are single and you are interested in tooling around and hoping to turn a few heads. A corvette might well do that. I can tell you that without a doubt that an old man in good shape on a bicycle will turn the heads of more thirty-five-year-old women who are tired of looking at their fat and out of shape husbands that you can shake a stick at. And you can save about $99K in the process.

Everyone likes being appreciated. Everyone likes being looked up to. As you get older, and God willing you shall, the better the physical condition you can maintain, the more benefits you will realize from that effort, physically, psychologically, economically, spiritually, and sexually. Damn near everything about your life gets better when you exercise. Even your kids will look up to you as they see the difference between other parents who don't exercise and you and the difference in appearance and capabilities.

Which brings us to another subject. We not only have a lot of overweight adults in this country, we have a lot of overweight kids. Many of you readers are at some point in the parenthood continuum. As you no doubt remember, whether it is now or was several years ago, having little kids watching you changes your behavior. You do this and you don't do that as a result of being watched by little humans whose trust in your credibility is imperative. Well guess what, having adult kids watching you is good for your behavior as well. One of the best things you can do for your kids is set an example that they should be proud to follow. An example that they cannot ridicule. An example that is not lame. This is not a book about how to deal with your kids. The only reason to bring it up is for the health and well-being of all concerned. It is also helpful in terms of time management, if your kids are involved in your exercise plans. My kids train with me at the martial arts dojo. It is a huge help in managing time, because we're around each other, we interact on the same subject, I can get my training in, and keep an eye on them at the same time. They are getting the same message about respect, discipline, and responsibility that my wife and I give them while they're getting exercise. I understand that your idea of physical recreation and your kids' idea of fun may not coincide. If you can find physically active things to do together you can solve several problems at once.

Another concept I'd like to bring up in relation to time management is sleep. Most people need between six and eight hours a night. If you watch any TV you will quickly come to the conclusion that a lot of people are not able to get a good night's sleep. When you see that many ads for medications to help you sleep, you know it is a common problem. Let me suggest an idea that may work for you. Earlier we talked about alternating workouts. One day I'll do my full workout and the next do a light one. On my light workout days I find it easier to wake up early and get my stretching and stick work in before the girls wake up. I'll sacrifice an hour of sleep to exercise and, in the process, I get better sleep in the remaining seven hours. It is common knowledge that regular exercise will help you get better quality sleep. You burn nervous energy, get a little physically tired, and work off aggression. Some sleep experts warn against exercising vigorously right before bedtime. The theory is that the increase in electrical activity in the brain will make it hard to fall asleep. I do not know about that, one way or another. If you elect to exercise right before bed, keep the possibility of encountering that problem in mind. It is very common behavior to spend the last hour or so of the day being a couch potato in front of the TV. If you can get off the couch and work out for a while you can squeeze in another couple of hours a week. Another way to squeeze another hour out of your day is to capture all the two to ten minute intervals that you spend waiting for something or someone. Before you try to actually use any of this new found time, first spend a week or so trying to identify it. Keep a little informal journal of the two minutes here and six minutes there that are presently idle, wasted time. You will be amazed at the end of the week what it adds up to. If you pay attention to this lost time it really adds up. Once you get used to recognizing these small periods of time, you will then prepare a plan for getting something useful out of them. If you are in full dress mode at the office you probably won't hit the deck and do a hundred sit-ups. What you can do is your hip and shoulder rotations or shoulder stretches or ankle lifts or squats. You get the idea. If you can keep your eyes open for those short periods of time and put them to good use, at the end of the week they've added up to another workout or two. You will have to get over feeling self- conscious about doing a few minutes of stretching or exercise in a non traditional setting. Uninformed people will look at you as if your behavior is a little weird. Oh, well. Most of those people would derive a lot of benefit from increasing their own   activity. Let me give you an analogy from way back in college. A great teacher named Fred McElroy gave me a really good tip early on in college. This professor recommended that his students take all the information from his physiology course that was required to be memorized and put it on three by five cards. He said, keep a stack of cards with you at all times and when you have two or ten minutes here or there during the day pull out your stack and go through them. He said, that way you won't have to devote an hour every night to memorization because you will already have done it throughout your day. Then you can spend that hour on math or chemistry or some non-memorization course. I did this with all my science courses that required memorization, and I routinely finished at or near the top of my class. I did not finish with good grades because I was so damn smart. It was because I had good advice and enough sense to pay attention to it and the willingness to work it. The same technique can be put to good use at fiftysomething. What about those times when you Just Don't Feel Like It! You have the time and you have the opportunity and you just don't feel like working out. Then don't. It's going to happen. If you are fortunate, those days will be rare. If you are on a pretty regular schedule of exercise and you want to play hooky now and then to do something else go ahead. It's like putting money in the bank. If you're working all the time you can afford to take a day off. I will skip a day here and there to go fishing. When I fish, I am in relaxation mode. When I work, when I train, and when I hunt, I work hard. When I fish, I relax. The kids have fun, I relax. Mission accomplished. Don't ever forget that the reason you are going to work this hard at staying in shape is to feel good and enjoy your health, enjoy your life. As the years progress, the demands on you will change. Kids and parents and payments and wants will all demand either more or less; only time will tell. Once you have established a base exercise regimen, especially if I can convince you to start training in the martial arts, you will be able to roll with the punches and adapt to the obstacles that life tosses in your path.

Dealing With Pain

One thing I am certain of is that I do not need to tell you that you are going to have to deal with pain. This you already know. Rare is the human who gets to the age of forty or fifty and does not have aches and pains. I have heard it said that growing old ain't for sissies. I am fifty-two and I have my share of little aches and pains. And on occasion, I have significant pain. There are a couple of things we need to consider as we approach how we are going to deal with pain. The first and foremost consideration is identifying your pain tolerance level and whether you need to change it. Or, perhaps more accurately, can you change it? No one can answer this but you. We all have to deal with and evaluate the minor pain we feel and decide. Is it a little ache that I can work through or is it an impending injury and I need to back off?

I'm going to give you a couple of general guideline examples and you will work forward in your analysis from there. On the one hand is the athlete who is so gung-ho to compete that he or she ignores the pain signals from the body until an injury is exacerbated to the point of being debilitating. Then they are forced to shut down. This usually happens to younger athletes who still consider themselves invincible and don't have a history of minor pains slowing them down. That mindset is seldom the case with older athletes. Most of us in our forties and fifties know that if you don't back off your workout in time when your knee is barking at you, you may not use it for a month. You have seen this before. On the other end of the spectrum is the person who uses every little condition of tightness and discomfort as an excuse to shut down and not work out. That is, unfortunately, the norm. So many people fall into this category that we have the sad state of physical condition in this country in which obesity has reached epidemic proportions. Only you can judge for yourself. In spite of what Ol' Bill would lead you to believe, only you can feel your pain. As you learn to deal with this dilemma of deciding which degree of pain is the little ache to work through and which is an impending injury that you should back off from, I have a plan for you. There is a really good chance that most every day, something is going to hurt. By pain I mean primarily the little aches and pains we all get. Some of them will be borderline in intensity and will make you uncertain as to your approach. Work through or back off? Well, the answer is easy. If in doubt, back off, do something else and then try again in about five minutes. If it hurts less, work through a bit. If that works, keep on going. If it still hurts a significant amount, back off for a few days. You will have so many different exercises to do by the time you get through this series that there is no way you will be able to get to all of them in a workout anyway. So if one day your elbow says that you are not doing push-ups today, you simply shift that time and effort to squats or calves or sit-ups or curls, et cetera. I have a herniated disk in my back at L5-S1. It is a pretty typical rupture with the disk tissue extruded and obliterating the nerve trunk. The MRI and the x-ray show a significant reduction in intervertebral space. When it first happened some seventeen years ago it was a severely debilitating injury. When I was working during the day, I was in excruciating pain a lot of the time. After work I would lie on the floor for relief. That went on for six months until I found a doctor who was able to provide me with relief. I had sought several opinions and examined different modalities of treatment during that time. None of them offered very good odds or a sound logical plan that I was willing to pursue. In the last seventeen years I have had only a couple of bouts of pain with recurring sciatica from the disk. My point is that you will have different levels of pain from minor twinges to debilitating injury and you will learn to work through them because the options may be pretty bleak. You have seen crippled up and invalid non-ambulatory people younger than you are. You will see them in their motorized carts at the store and you do not want this to happen to you if there is any way you can avoid it. Odds are really good that you can. You would not be reading this book if that were not the case. Chances are that if you are unfortunate enough to sustain a significant injury you will know it. You will then seek out the various doctors to get opinions, then decide on treatment and hope for the best. The little aches and pains that you will learn to work through will require lots of self- management. The exercises you are learning here will do more than anything else to reduce your pain. Beyond that there are a few simple concepts to learn that will help you understand and manage minor pain.

As we age our tissues become less supple. Typically we lose a significant amount of range of motion because our day-to-day routine does not cause us to maintain what we were blessed with at the age of sixteen. As we engage in activities at fifty-something, a couple of things happen. First we will get minor strains of our muscle tissue, connective tissue, and joints. These strains amount to microscopic tears in the fabric of the tissue. You can think of most of your connective tissues, the tendons and ligaments, as similar to a sheet of ropelike material. When you are young you can jerk the rope around, give it a good pull, no problem. When you are older you must be more careful with putting sudden strain on the rope. If you warm it up it works quite well. Without warm-up it may be quite stiff. When a fifty-something person experiences pain in a tendon or muscle it is very often a minor strain that for all intents and purposes amounts to a microscopic tear in the fiber of that tissue. That is not as bad as it sounds. As you have read in the Flexibility and Range of Motion section, the stretching of tissue requires microscopic tearing of that tissue. As you work your tissues, muscle, connective and bone, you will get some inflammation. This goes along with the microscopic tears we call strains. Anti-inflammatory medications will be a valuable asset in dealing with the attendant pain. You are already familiar with most of these medications. They are from the NSAID group, the non-steroidal anti-inflammatory group of medications. The kind of stuff you take for a headache will help with any pain associated with your workouts. Again, when you repeatedly contract muscle tissue and stretch connective tissue you are causing microscopic tears in that tissue. That tissue will repair itself in a thicker, stronger, and longer shape, which is good. That is the reason for your workout. In the process you will get a little inflammation associated with the process. This is where the anti-inflammatory medications can be of great help. They interrupt the chemistry of the inflammation and help shut it down. As a result, they lessen the pain. Now NSAIDS are not without their side effects and are not to be taken carelessly. They are a very useful adjunct in our desire to obtain the healthful results of an active life. Any time you have a significant enough injury to a joint to require a steroidal injection, you will no doubt be resting that joint for an extended period of time. You will know, and your doctor will tell you, that you over did it. Avoiding injury from over-training is particularly important to us older people as we do not bounce back as fast as we used to. And that is pretty much it. I could go into a whole bunch of scientific details and specific explanations of studies and trends and tissue samples and fill several pages with it. The end result would be a longer and no more useful book.

Productivity

One of the most common excuses that is offered up a reason for lack of exercise is time and cost constraints. A person will claim that they cannot find the time as doing so would mean working less and losing income. There is no time to take away from the kids and every available hour is occupied by fruitful gain or asset maintenance. Well that may be true and it may be achievable for a while, but somewhere around the age of forty, that argument begins to lose its legs. Or should I say, peter out, run out of gas. Go soft. Somewhere around forty as most non-exercisers begin to run out of energy, those who have a fitness plan, like the you will learn about here, will tell you how the increase in productivity they enjoy as a result of their fitness far outpaces the costs involved. Such numbers are absolutely impossible to quantify with any accuracy.

I can assure you that after complete fitness training becomes a way of life you will attest to the improvement in your productivity. It may be as simple as your ability to perform various tasks at a more efficient pace. You get offered a better job opportunity because you are fit. You may be perceived as a lower risk to a potential employer or business partner. You may benefit from being more pleasant to look at. You will be held in higher esteem as a result of being truly physically fit at an age where most people have thrown in the towel. I have the perfect example. Me. I started working out at a pretty good clip about four years ago at the age of forty-eight. I have refined and adjusted over time. I have been going out of my way to avoid home improvement projects for a couple of years now. I tightened up my schedule at the office to make sure I get out early on Tuesday and Thursday for big workout days. On weekends there is plenty of time to exercise, no excuses. I can absolutely tell you that my productivity at work is better than it would be if I was in the same shape as the guy next door.

And get this: I have the opportunity to put the knowledge into a form that will benefit you. You will look at this information and say, "Yes, I'll pay twelve or forty or one hundred dollars to learn this because I will benefit a thousand times over as a result of doing the stuff that's in here." Once you learn the information and training techniques in this series you are done spending money here. You can then actually make money doing this, not to mention the money and time you will save on medical costs and procedures as a result of the improvements you will see in your health. And, of course, there is the increase in productivity you will experience as a result of the improvement of your physical condition. Can you imagine in real dollars how much it would cost you to have cardiac bypass surgery because you could not find the time to exercise? There are certain absolutely legitimate tax deductible opportunities that I became aware of even before I sold my first book or DVD. You might very well be able to find the same. When you get in good enough shape to start teaching fitness you might find you can gain from tax-deductible travel and dojo or gym dues as well as laundry and clothing allowances. You get my drift. Ironic as it may sound, there is one excuse for not exercising that I can relate to. I sometimes use it myself. "I just don't feel like it". It happens. To me, it happens about one out of ten exercise opportunities. And I probably opt out of the workout about half of the time. So every now and then I have an opportunity to get ten to thirty minutes of some beneficial activity in and I just don't feel like it. Oh, well.

STRESS

I do not need to tell you what stress is. You have enough of it in your life to be able to define it yourself, of this I am sure. Most of us have believed, for most of our lives, that stress is something to avoid. To a large extent this is probably good advice. There are a lot of forms of stress that are not healthy and not good for us, both on a physical as well as a psychological level. The results and ramifications of unresolved stress can result in exhaustion, pain, tissue damage, loss of sleep, addiction, damage to your relationships, you name it. Stress as a concept has been around a long time, probably since the beginning of intelligent life on earth. Shakespeare has a passage in one of his plays regarding "the flailing of arms and the gnashing of teeth." These represent unfavorable and negative responses to stress.

There are a few examples of stresses that can be deemed as beneficial stresses. This category is defined more by our responses to them than the stress itself. If you are eighteen, you may think about the need for money to buy a house and a car and support a family you hope to have one day. This could motivate you to excel in school; this is a good stress and response situation. If you have anxiety about feeling run-down and lacking energy and you are staring down the barrel of your fortieth birthday and you use that stress to workout with this program, then that is good stress. There are some forms of stress that life imposes upon us that we can not avoid and all you can do is deal with them. There are others that are self-imposed, self-inflicted and we'll do our best to learn to recognize them and get rid of them, or at least deal with them in a healthy manner. I once heard a great quote. When I was a kid, there was a golfer named Lee Trevino. He had just finished a round in a tournament and a reporter asked him if he felt stress at having to sink a particular putt. His answer was that, no, that wasn't stress. Stress is when you are down to your last fifteen dollars. Trevino was playing a round of golf that might have been worth a $100,000 to him and yet he recognized the difference between that magnitude of money and the dollars that really matter. As people, we do these sorts of miscalculations all the time. We often misjudge the importance of things to accrue versus activities that matter. One of the problems that come with the mind set of desiring acquisitions is that things cost money. The money you must earn to pay the price costs you time and effort. Don't forget that you pay taxes on that coin as well. Many of the things to do also have costs involved. A lot of them are relatively small. Doing push-ups costs you only a few minutes. No dollars and no taxes. And the effort relieves stress. More on that later.

So let us take a little look at stress, the good and the bad. We will surely be able to spend a lot more time talking about bad stress and what to do about it, so let's start by looking at some of the good things about stress. I know this may seem redundant, but it really does deserve repeating. I hope you will spend a few moments each day examining the stresses placed on you and deciding that you can do without some of them. If you have an impending deadline. If you have a goal in your future and in order to accomplish that goal you need to set yourself on a course of preparation, you will feel the pressure of a timetable. If you do not start preparing tomorrow and stick to your schedule for the next four months you will not excel at the biochemistry exam. If you do not stretch diligently and work on your spinning side kick and redondo stick technique, you will not look good for your brown belt test. If you do not answer your alarm and get to work on time you will not be able to put food on the table for your children. These are examples of relatively good kinds of stresses. You have a worthwhile objective, a plan of action, and a reasonable chance of success. These kinds of stresses you can productively act on in a positive manner and they do not have a great deal of accompanying anxiety. They may have some anxiety, but hopefully not much. Some of that depends on your degree of self-confidence. For the most part, if you prepare, you have a reasonable expectation of success. Another example of how this kind of stress can be good comes when you consider your long-term future. Say you are fifty and you would like to be able to still go elk hunting when you are eighty. If the fear and stress of being immobile and decrepit at an early age gets you to workout a little bit more, then that is good stress.

Bad stress. Life delivers plenty of that. Some of the stress life delivers to you can't be helped and you just have to figure how to deal with it. It is very easy and very common for people to want to buy too much car and too much house. Some of this mindset is driven by advertising; in the early 2000s it was aided by low interest rates. When rates increase, affordability wanes and a lot of stress ensues. Something that fifty-somethings must grasp if they are to enjoy their remaining years on this earth, and hopefully teach their kids, is that more is not always better. Sometimes it is and sometimes it is not.

One aspect of this stress related analysis that I see a lot of as a practicing dentist is Shakespeare's adage of the flailing of arms and the gnashing of teeth. We touched on this earlier. It bears repeating. A lot of people grind and clench their teeth as a response to unresolved stress. This is not just my opinion. This is the reasoned analysis of psychologists and is something I have seen several times each week for the last 25 years. The grinding of teeth, either during the day or at night, can do a lot of damage to the teeth and jaw. It can also cause a lot of pain. In severe cases, it can predispose the patient to temporal mandibular joint syndrome[TMJ]. This can be a physically debilitating set of maladies related to dysfunction of the TMJ. People with this syndrome get headaches of great magnitude, vision disruption, nausea, and dizziness.

People who are forced to or force themselves to live under undo stress are more likely to suffer heart disease, ulcers in their stomach, irritable bowel syndrome, and a host of other problems. One advantage to being fifty is that there is a good chance you have learned some good coping mechanisms for dealing with stress by now. Many good methods of dealing with stress involve not letting it occur in the first place. Sometimes it does not matter what our defenses are. Exercise is one of the very best things you can do to burn off the anxiety that comes with stress. Again, I am talking about regular exercise of the type you are learning about in this series. When you know you have a regular workout scheduled (and it is even better if there is bag work involved), stressful events do not have a chance to pile up on you. You know you have an opportunity to vent coming at five o'clock. You are going to the dojo and kick the crap out of a wavemaster. And you will feel better. In terms of fitness and health, you certainly know that stress causes increases in blood pressure and stomach acid as well as anxiety-related bad decisions, nervous eating, and on and on. So stick to your workouts. Burn off the stress before it affects you.

Life is too short to allow the bad stuff to be amplified. If you intend to live and love in this life you will be forced to pay a price for it. God willing, I hope you will never have to undergo the unimaginable suffering of losing a child. If you get to live to be old, as we all hope we will, you will lose your parents and a few friends and if you are lucky you will lose a good dog or two. I say lucky because of the unfortunate fact that dogs live relatively short lives. And life is not full without a good dog.

My wife and I are dog people, as in "god" spelled backwards. As of this writing, Marshall is thirteen years old. His kidneys are failing and his arthritis makes it hard for him to move around. He is one of the most handsome black Labradors you could ever lay eyes on. He's not got a speck of grey on him. As he sits up, you would think he is five. It was only a couple of short years ago that we were hunting pheasants and quail and ducks and geese. Marshy would work methodically. Reliably. From the time we got out of the truck until the day was done. Some days I would miss bird after bird and he never once gave me a look of "What's the matter dude? Can't shoot straight?" He would just get back to work, looking for the next bird. And as luck would have it, we'd hit three in a row and he would bring them to me and with the wag of his tail, tell me I did well. When he was young I would feed him a cheeseburger after a hard days work. I do not know if it is important to think about dietary constraints for dogs like people need to, other than for concerns about obesity. Marshy will not hunt this year. Hopefully his kidneys will carry him through another year. Either way, he will not be with us much longer. By the time you read this he will likely be gone. And we will cry for the loss of a good dog.

Last year we lost Simon. He was a Lab and Dalmatian mix. He developed a cancer in his foreleg and lasted six months. He was a clown. When he was young I would not have given you a plug nickel for him. My wife brought him home after a moment of weakness. She went to the pet store to get a new collar for Marshall as he was growing and there was Simon, crying and yelping "take me home:" Since I had been drinking, I let him in the door and named him. As a result he was mine. He was no smarter than a carrot and exasperated me to no end as I tried to teach him the very simple obligations that a dog has in our family. Needless to say, he did not hunt. But he was a part of our family, so he stayed. And he did one of the most remarkable things over the almost eleven years that he lived. He got smarter. I have had several Labs in the last thirty years and some have lived long and tragedy has taken a few to young. All of my labs were pretty smart animals and at a relatively young age demonstrated that they could figure out what I asked of them. That was not the case with Simon. What Simon did was more remarkable. Each and every year he lived he got a little smarter to the program we expect from the dogs at our house, and he turned into a real good dog in the process. This is a human attribute. Most of my more intelligent dogs rose to their height of intellectual capacity early on in life and stayed there.

Any modicum of human intelligence will cause you to act smarter as you age. The acquisition of wisdom is one of the absolutely best things about growing older. Sadly very few people manage a whole bunch. I am not saying it is rare, but it certainly isn't common. That is probably one of the two biggest reasons, well three, that most youngsters don't listen to their elders. The elders are not all that wise; their intellectual capacity was never large, or they were blinded by greed or poverty or fear or you name it.

A big part of being fit at fifty-something involves getting smarter as you get older. You have to keep yourself out of trouble by taking a moment longer to assess the path ahead prior to hurrying down it. You have the discipline to be methodical and perseverant. One of the attributes present in almost all the people I have met who are over fifty and truly physically fit is the ability to remind themselves to take full advantage of every opportunity to work exercise into their schedule. Even if it is only five minutes of tai chi here and there or five minutes of breathing exercises. Like saving your pocket change in a bucket, you can or trim a hundred calories by eating two veggies with your pasta and ribs. Try a ripe nectarine instead of ice cream for dessert. But you knew that already. Addition by subtraction. Most of this stuff is so simple, it obligates me to keep this book short. I could go on and on with examples and description and direction about the micromanagement of your diet and your financial acquisition strategy and workload, but it would probably do little good. The truths that you find or deny in the process of figuring what you will do with the last three-eights of your life are for you to decide. You most certainly will not be following me anywhere. What will be notable in the thirty or so years you have left is whether you try to do something remarkable and respectable with that time or something normal and pedantic. There are so many physical, psychological, and social advantages gained by the fifty-something who maintains true physical fitness that you simply cannot afford to give it less than your best effort. Spend a good part of the next week looking around at the people you see. Look at the average physical condition of the forty- to fifty- to sixty- year-old people you see. Hopefully you will decide that you do not want to look and feel like most of those you see.

SEX: LOOKING GOOD AND BETTER WOOD

You cannot possibly turn on your TV and watch a complete show without seeing an advertisement for a medication to treat ED. Now I am fifty-two and I can tell that those ads are aimed straight at me. The only reason that the pharmaceutical companies spend that much money on so many TV ads is they know there are lots and lots of fifty-something guys out here who need help getting it up; the profit per pill is good. I am glad that these meds are available. I have had the good fortune in not yet needing any. That doesn't mean I won't next year. This subject of sex and physical attractiveness is so important; it dominates our culture to a completely disproportionate level. Most young people are so concerned about their looks they might even be willing to exercise and adopt a healthy diet to look good. Just kidding. We have more fat adolescents than ever. Turns out many of those fat and unattractive adolescents resort to submissive and self-degrading sexual behavior in order to be temporarily desired by their peers. All the more reason to exercise, teach your kids to exercise, and eat healthy. Help them develop the self-esteem to feel good about themselves and not have to resort to submissive behavior to be desired. Setting an example of healthy exercise patterns for your kids will motivate them to develop desirable and respected habits. But I digress.

It is true that a fraction of our society's population is willing to make the effort to get healthy and enjoy the rewards that come from that effort. Since you are reading this book, there is a good chance you are one of them. Sex, sex, sex. Chances are that at fifty-something you don't need as much as you did when you were young. Or at least you're not thinking about it all the time the way you were. Based on the current rate of advertising buys, there are a lot of guys out there who want to have more and better sexual performance and are willing to spend the cash on an ED medication to make it happen. Now it is absolutely normal that as males age their sexual potency should wane. Let's go back to our examination of human history and the evolution of the human animal. Up until a couple of hundred years ago the life expectancy of a human didn't extend much beyond forty years. The drive to reproduce was strongest in the late teen and early twenty-year range. This is the period of greatest physical strength and it gave the parents time to raise a child to the age of fourteen or so, when they were candidates to begin reproduction and repeat the cycle. I am not sufficiently trained in psychology to make a definitive claim. However I suspect the reason that female sexual drive peaks nearer to forty is the ticking of the clock phenomenon. This repetition of the cycle of reproduction is what has defined success for generations of all species. In the last two hundred years things have really changed for the human animal -society, medicine, education, wealth. Yet physically our bodies are almost identical to the human form of several thousand years ago. So now we find ourselves in a time when it often takes until the age of twenty-five to become educated and a few more years to actually start making significant amounts of money. The next thing you know you are thirty- something before you start having kids. Before you know it, you are forty and it becomes more difficult to reproduce. Women are up against a bunch of daunting statistics from forty on. The formula kind of stinks. You finally get to an age where you can afford to pay for the costs of having a homestead and you're running out of time for the greatest joy and burden of life, being a parent. If you suffer any difficulties in reproduction, you can find that time runs out on you very quickly. Most of the reproductive issues regarding birth defects and age you can do nothing to change. The only way to try to avoid them is to have kids at a younger age, in your twenties instead of your thirties (or forties as some of us nitwits have done). I make the statement as the numero uno nitwit in this regard.

Again I digress. So let's get back to what we started talking about at the outset, which is basically that we want to have recreational sex on a regular basis. It does not matter if we are twenty, thirty, forty, or fifty-something. We want to enjoy it, we want our partner to enjoy it, and be thinking about it tomorrow, and when am I going to get some more? Again, for you fifty-somethings, we're done having kids, right? Now let's just fornicate for the fun of it! So, a large part of the drive to reproduce is over. Your time has past. Most of you women have good enough sense to know that reproduction is likely to be problematical when they are much past forty. Most of us idiot males get it by fifty. So now a lot of the reproductive urgency and biologic drive is gone. Now we can get down to having fun. We are going to talk about a couple of things here.

That just reminded me of a joke. Do you know why men can't get mad cow disease? Because we're pigs!

Males are visual animals. I do not know why. But I know it is true. Men look at a female form of big tits, slim waist, and a nice butt and are imbued with a visceral feeling of desire. Now if your mother taught you well, you behave in a socially acceptable manner when it comes to that desire, which means you keep it to yourself or maybe talk about it with your buddies. You can look at theories of large breasts being a harbinger of milk production for offspring, I do not know. I do know that there were very few fat females up until the last fifty years or so. Why that model is universally considered visually repulsive to males I do not know. I just know that it is. Before I became a husband and father to daughters I was no different. To some extent I still am no different. I am fortunate in that my wife works out and looks good and visually I am pleased. As I am fifty-two, I pray she tells me we are done having kids. So let's get back to the subject of what are we going to do to be able to have wild raucous sex well into old age. Well, we may not be so robust on the wild and raucous part but we can still keep going for a long time. A message for you guys out there. The very same exercise that strengthens your heart and endurance is going to directly apply to providing you with better wood. Exercise strengthens your heart and improves blood flow. Your penis is largely comprised of a corpus spongiosum tissue that requires vascular engorgement to achieve and maintain a mutually satisfactory erection. Eminent cardiologists such as Dr Mehmet Oz have long made the correlation between cardiovascular health and male sexual performance. For you guys, there is nothing more important that you can do for strengthening your ability to have a satisfactory erection than working out. Working out may also allow you to recapture enough of your health to be able to reduce some of the medications you may be taking. There are several medications that can exacerbate erectile dysfunction. Working out will make you look better. This will make your partner enjoy looking at you more. This will enhance your ego, and your libido, on and on.

Girls, the very same news that seems completely unfair turns out to be your biggest stick. Reproduction is a female burden. I mean physically. I can hear you now "tell me something I don't know." If men had to carry babies there would be no children. If you reproduce with a responsible male who agrees to pay for the costs and help with child- rearing then you don't get saddled with the entire effort. Facts is facts, and physically, females produce offspring. It is absolutely and perfectly normal for a pregnant female to eat. A lot. After the child is born, there is likely to be residual weight gain. From a health and aesthetic viewpoint, most new moms would like to lose that extra weight, which is not easy. But it can be done. Let's assume that you are beyond your reproductive years. From here on out you will no longer be subjecting your body to the hormonal and emotional roller coaster of reproduction. You did what you did, you are where you are. Again, let me guess that you are at least forty-something and maybe fifty or so. I kid you not when I tell you that if you do your exercise regimen and get yourself in the best possible shape, your old fart will respond. In this manner you will re-exert a tremendous amount of control over the situation which is, of course, what you want. In almost every species, the female controls reproduction. In the case of humans, it also means the female controls recreational sex. When environmental conditions are right, the female comes into estrus and the male is programmed to respond. He can't help it. Unless something is wrong. Again, male humans are visual animals. If you provide the bait and drag it through the water you will get a strike. Sad but true, males have little more control than a pea-brained fish. We men are just that predictable, weak, helpless, and simple. I know. I am one. Again, I am probably not telling you ladies anything you do not already know. It reminds me of a Robert Cray song " It's easy to see but It's hard to admit.".The point it that you gals have control over males well into your fifties. Do not worry about a few wrinkles and you don't need to spend a lot of money on all the creams and moisturizer products and age defying potions on TV. Work out and control your diet and the male or males in your life will see the difference and respond. We can't help it.

INFLAMMATION

The subject of inflammation is one that has recently seen a tremendous increase of scientific inquiry. As a practicing dentist, I cannot be happier to see this occur. When new patients come to me and present themselves with a mouthful of maladies, the dental disease that I see and treat has a component of inflammation about ninety percent of the time. Medical doctors, especially cardiologists, have become aware in the last few years of how harmful chronic inflammation can be. I am not going to bore you with the biochemistry of inflammation, but it is important and valuable that you have a working knowledge of the process. When your tissue is afflicted with either infection or trauma, inflammation will occur. If you are damaged or invaded in any way, inflammation is a part of the healing process. If you experience any sort of bruise or tear to your tissue, whether it is a bump or a scratch, your body will initiate the inflammatory response. For the most part this is good; it is the beginning of the biochemical process of healing. Inflammation is the body's little siren to call in the defenses and start the process of killing the bacterial or viral invaders and /or rebuilding the tissue that was damaged by traumatic injury. Inflammation has probably been a component of human tissue for as long as humans have been around, 100,000 years or so, give or take. So it is nothing new, it is just that our understanding of it that is improving.

As a dentist, I see ten to fifteen patients a day. Depending on the condition of their mouth, each person may have little to no inflammation present, or they may have a significant amount of inflammation present. I know I am at risk of getting boring but stay with me because I promise you the information will be worth it. The human mouth is about as perfect a place as you could devise for growing bacteria. It is warm. It is wet, and you throw food in it. A similar analogy would be if you squirted a little water into your garbage can every day in July. Since you have a service to empty your garbage can, you only need to open it to throw stuff in. Chances are you stand back and do not breathe as you throw. You get the picture. If you are in the habit of cleaning your mouth thoroughly twice a day, and that means brushing and flossing twice a day, then pat yourself on the back. For you are in the minority. The bacteria that live in your mouth form a layer of plaque on your teeth on about a twenty four hour cycle. That means if you brush and floss today, tomorrow you will have a layer of plaque on any surface that you did not physically, mechanically wipe clean. That layer of plaque is the nest that the bacteria build for itself on the surface of your teeth. Don't fall asleep. This is useful. Remember the shot! Plaque is like a fishing net folded over on itself and the bacteria live in the holes in the net. And they wait to be fed. And they eat whenever you eat. Their favorite food is sugar. You feed them sugar and it is party time! They eat the sugar, they metabolize, and they excrete. What they excrete is primarily acid, and other toxic byproducts. The acid dissolves the calcium of the tooth and starts the formation of a cavity. If this pattern continues, and it does, the bacteria invade the tooth and a cavity forms. A cavity is an infection of the mineralized tissue of the tooth. So what. you say, everyone gets cavities! Can you get done with this boring subject? Yes I can. And I will. When I am finished! So be quiet and listen. This is important. Not just to avoid cavities and periodontal [gum] disease. The infection that starts in a tooth will progress to the nerve of the tooth and on to the supporting bone. None of which you want happening to you.

The cardiologists have come to the conclusion that the inflammation in your mouth can be as big a risk factor for heart disease as smoking tobacco, hypertension, stress, obesity, lack of exercise, high cholesterol and stress and on an on. You have known for a long time what to do and not do for cardiac health. If you were young, you barely paid attention. If you engaged in unhealthy cardiac behavior, you probably barely paid attention or lived in denial.

There are a couple of good reasons for going through the exercise of teaching you about cavities and periodontal disease. If you have a modicum of intelligence and your head even halfway out of the sand, you want to pay heed to a really easy, painless, inexpensive, and convenient way to avoid disease, defect and debilitation in an area of your body that will have a direct effect on your health well into your old age. What do you imagine happens to an elderly tiger when he loses his teeth? He dies. Worse than that, he dies of starvation. Most people can barely stand being hungry long enough to avoid obesity. What happens to an elderly human when he loses his teeth? He gets dentures. And then he dies of starvation. Sure he can eat, we dentists are pretty good at making a set of teeth that can chew a lot of stuff, but denture wearers cannot eat all foods. Denture wearers suffer a degree of malnutrition as a result of their inability to chew. There is a lot of nutrition they miss out on. Many of the fresh fruits and veggies and the nuts and seeds get left out of the diet because it hurts when they get under a denture. My point is that you should not neglect your teeth. Keep them as healthy as you can and they will help you remain as healthy as you can be in your old age.

In your mouth, if you leave bacteria and plaque on a tooth surface, the inflammation that results from that infection causes the bone of your jaw to degrade. The cells that build and breakdown bone have enzymatic machinery that can run in both directions, depending on the stimuli they receive. If you put tension on bone it will build. If you put pressure on bone, or expose it to inflammation in the gum, or if the cardiac muscle demands calcium, bone will break down. It is the jawbone that holds on to the root of the tooth and makes it strong. If you lose that supporting bone, you cannot get it back.

You know the old saying in real estate - "location, location, location." In dental health, it's "prevention, prevention, prevention." And prevention costs you very few dollars and very few minutes of your time. Most people will do a pretty good job of brushing their teeth and not so good a job of flossing. They have it ingrained in their head to brush twice a day. I have seen countless numbers of people over the years who have shied away from flossing because they have been taught a very elaborate and time-consuming technique of wrapping the floss around the side of each tooth etc.. etc. I tell people it should not take more than twenty seconds to floss their entire mouth. All they need do is a quick up and down through the contact point between the teeth. Frequency is what counts. Floss your teeth. Twice a day. Every day. Save yourself a ton of grief. Eliminate the inflammation that is present in your mouth. It is good for your heart.

Balance Control

Maintaining your balance. As in not falling down. Kinda important. Most of us who have hit the big FIVE-O have been introduced to the experience of turning suddenly and feeling that momentary disorientation that takes us just a second to regain complete balance control. Most of us have seen a senior citizen(which we aren't quite yet, but we can see it coming) turn and temporarily lose their sense of balance or orientation. You may have the same sense of loss of ability to turn your head, perhaps obvious when you backup your car. As far as I can tell it just comes with age. Fortunately there is something you can do about it. Most of the training on maintaining balance is relatively difficult to convey through the written word. As you examine and utilize the section on endurance you will find a lot of useful information on how to maintain control of your balance as the years go by. This is one area of your training in which it really behooves you to get the video series. It is very easy to show on the video and we do so. There are various exercises that are of the dual-purpose variety, they work on endurance and balance at the same time. I know this can sound like a shameless promotion of a product line that requires you to buy the next in a series if you want to keep up. That is not the case. Remember that we are attempting to convey to you, the knowledge of how to improve and maintain your health through your hard work. Some of that knowledge is physical and is best learned by watching and listening at the same time. Be sure to notice that the videos are priced relatively low, as compared to other exercise videos on the market. Part of that is due to the fact that I am the author, subject, and videographer, and we do not have to mark up the price to cover paying studio costs. I promise you this. The health benefits you will derive from utilizing the information on these videos will pay for themselves in actual dollars a thousand fold. What I mean is this: the increased productivity that you will realize in your dollar generating capacity as a result of the improvement in your health. Not to mention how much better you are going to feel. And look. Did I mention the sex?

Back to the subject of balance. Most people at fifty are not terribly concerned about losing their balance. Most people at eighty are petrified of it. What we want to do is learn, starting at fifty, how to maintain control of our balance so that somewhere in our seventies we need not live in fear of falling down. Do you remember the old saying "When you are sixty you fall down and break your hip, and when you are seventy you break your hip and fall down?" Well, what you are going to do with this series is put a stop to all of that. You are not going to break your hip. Speaking of hips, we are talking about one of my favorite anatomical subject areas. As you will ascertain as you read through this book and watch the attendant videos, I will be constantly trying to convince you to seek training in the martial arts. When it comes to balance control, flexibility, range of motion, muscular strength, endurance, confidence walking down the street, weight control, containment of fear, martial arts' training cannot be beat. And get this, we are going to teach you how to fall down and not get hurt in the process. You will learn to fall frontwards, backwards and sideways and roll out of it so that when you fall (and you will, sometime), you don't get hurt.

Don't forget there are a multitude of different martial arts out there that have been developed by various cultures. In the process of finding fun and rewarding physical activities to do, I'll keep nudging you to look at the martial arts. The dojo is the place where you train. If you walk into one dojo and it doesn't seem right for you, walk out and check out another one. I have been exposed to a wide variety of martial arts and I can tell you that there are some I like a lot and some I do not care to do. I really enjoy tae kwon do, which is primarily kicking and hip flexibility. I spend a lot of time on kenpo, which is made up of practical self-defense striking and blocking techniques. Both of these styles have a great deal of important applications for maintaining personal safety. . The third art I so enjoy is arnis, the filipino art of fighting with rattan cane sticks. This is so much fun; I hope you get a chance to try it. Arnis is a great defense for women to learn, because it enables the athlete to really smack a much larger man with those sticks. We fifty-somethings can really put the hurt on a younger assailant with a pair of sticks. Plus, it is something you can use as a weapon of self-defense when you are very old. And they are very convenient to keep with you. Say you are eighty-five, and your legs will not allow you to kick someone on either side of the head, like you could when you were fifty-five. If you can swing a stick, you can dispatch, dissuade, disable, and discourage a potential assailant into looking for an easier target. Did I mention that they are a lot of fun? When I was a kid I used to love playing baseball. I studied the game. I listened to my beloved San Francisco Giants play darned near 162 games a year. Well, 154 when I was real little. For me, baseball is a radio game. Lon Simmons and Hank Greenwald made the field come to life in my mind's eye. I watched and listened to Mays, Macovey, Marichal, and Hart. Mostly, I loved hitting baseballs. I realized in high school that if I could not hit a curve ball, I was not going to make it to the bigs. I was not going to replace Mays in center field for the Giants. This was one of the early major disappointments in a young man's life. The importance of academic achievement became amplified. I have been going to the batting cages off and on over the years, just for the fun of hitting baseballs. It is good exercise as well as excellent eye/hand coordination activity. The same is true of stick work. When you train in arnis, the mental aspects of targeting and fast motion, with eye/hand coordination, are really invigorating. And having the ability to defend yourself simply cannot be overrated! I hope you get to try it.

Breathing

When it comes to being taken for granted, breathing has to rank right up at the top. It is even higher up than the people who pay all the taxes. It is one of those things that is taken completely for granted, a given, without thought. Until it is taken away. And it does not take long. The moment you can't breathe, it quickly becomes very important. Consider how many times a day you breathe, without ever giving it any thought, you inconsiderate lout. I'm going to give you a few tips about breathing that were taught to me. These will go a long way toward keeping your workouts aerobic as opposed to anaerobic, and help you as a relaxation technique as well.

Like most other people, you may have taken part in some form of aerobic fitness activity, jogging or bicycling or swimming. You have probably noticed that as you engage in the exercise, you started breathing faster and deeper. As you performed the effort, your body demanded more oxygen. Pretty simple. For repetitive motion exercises, you usually do not have a problem with the breathing rate keeping up with the demand. As you are running along, if you can keep up a light conversation between breaths, you are probably moving at the right pace. If you are breathing at a rate during which you cannot talk, you are pushing things at a pace you can maintain only for a short while. If you can chatterbox, then you probably need to step it up a bit.

During your aerobic training and/or endurance training, you probably won't have too much problem with oxygen load. Some types of exercises are accompanied by a tendency to hold your breath. For me, sparring is one activity during which I really have to pay attention to my breathing to make certain I do not cut short my wind by holding my breath. It took quite a while for me to recognize and correct my breath-holding tendencies during sustained efforts. The kiai is a great tool to remind your body to breathe. You have heard that shout martial artists make when they break a board. Tennis is another sport where you move quickly to another position and make a significant effort once you get there. This is similar to sparring in the martial arts. Tennis players often grunt at each shot. This forced expulsion of air is a mechanism to get the body to breathe in. Think of the kiai in karate, the grunt in tennis. Don't cut yourself short on air.

There is another aspect of breathing that I want to tell you about, one that I want you to practice for a few minutes each day. If you really feel you benefit from the relaxation this provides, you certainly can do a lot more. Lie on your back. With your arms at your sides, spread them out to about halfway to perpendicular to your body. As you breathe in, try to push your navel up to the ceiling as you fill your lungs to their absolute capacity. Breathe in at a rate that takes you about six seconds to completely fill your lungs. Next, expel the air at a rate that takes about eight seconds to empty your lungs. Try to push your navel against the floor in the process. Repeat and repeat. You will find this very relaxing. It is a technique in many training regimens, such as yoga, tai chi, karate, et cetera. There is not a whole lot more on the subject of fitness for me to add. Again, my tendency is to keep things simple. You can certainly continue reading from various other sources on the subjects of nutrition and flexibility and sleep and meditation and on and on. You will undoubtedly find nuggets of knowledge that will complement what I have offered here. Go explore. Add to your knowledge base. Don't forget to stretch.

FLEXIBILITY AND RANGE OF MOTION EXERCISES

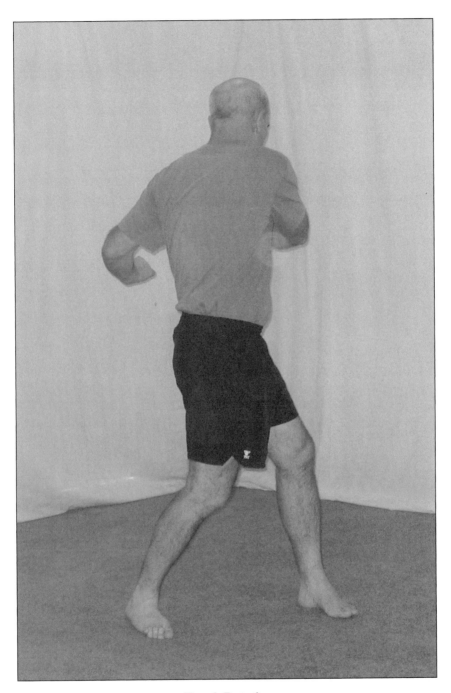

Trunk Rotation

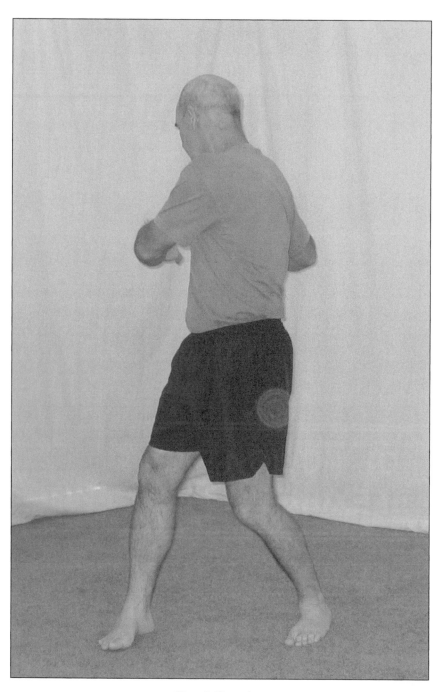

Trunk Rotation

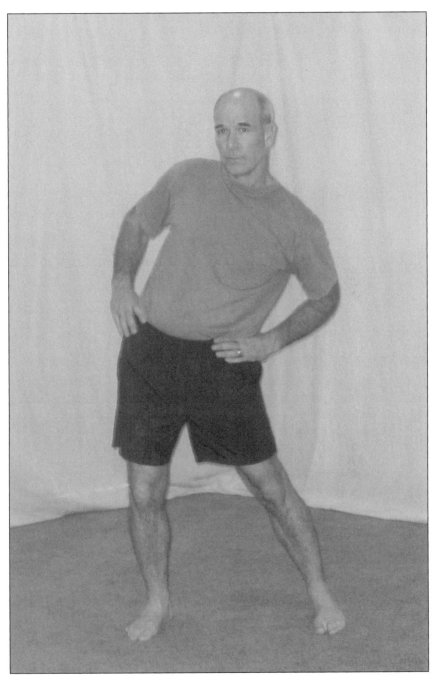

Hip Rotation

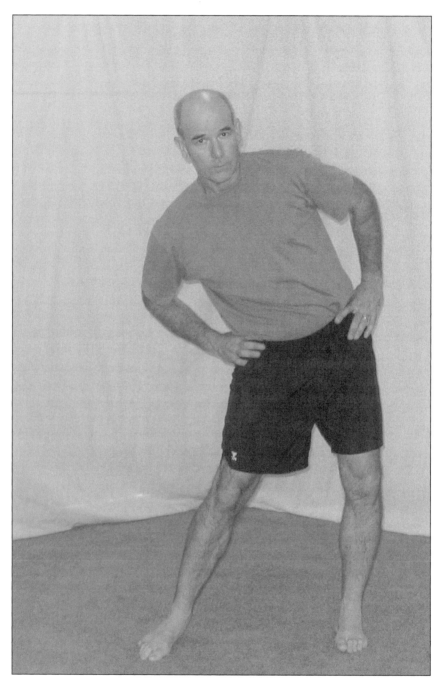

Hip Rotation

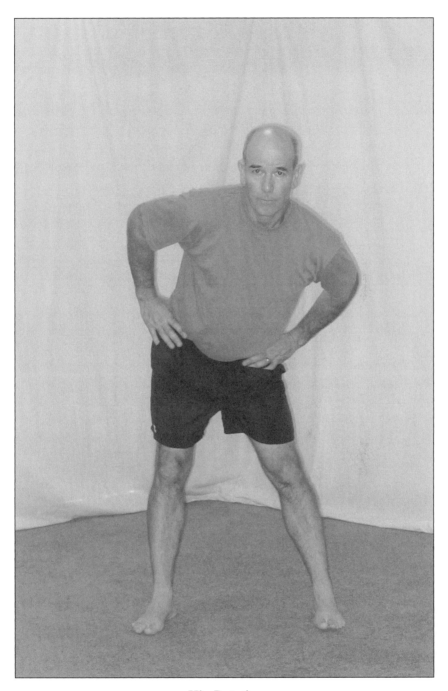

Hip Rotation

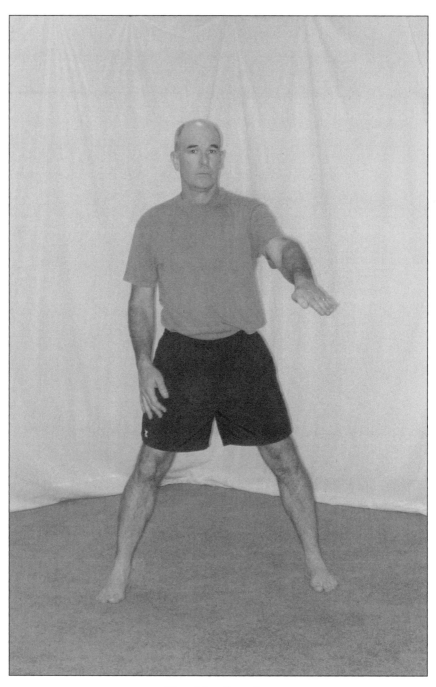

Shoulder Rotation

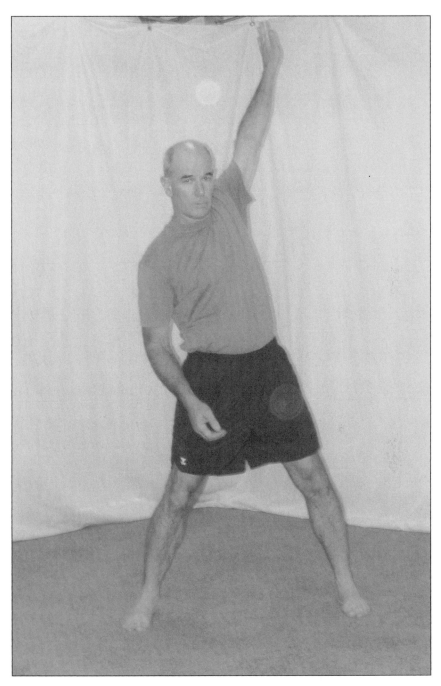

Shoulder Rotation

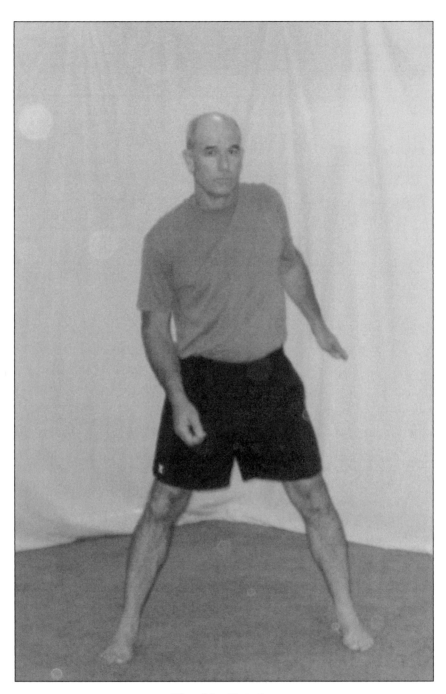

Shoulder Rotation

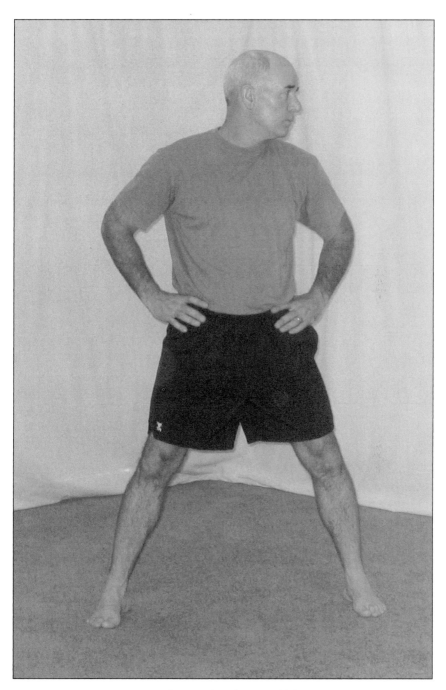

Neck Rotation Side to Side

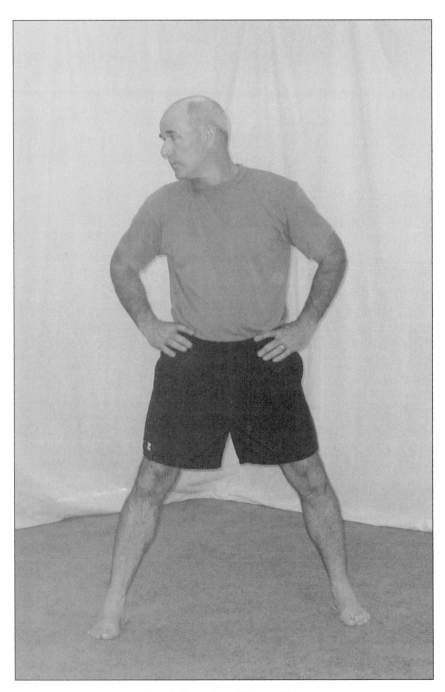

Neck Rotation Side to Side

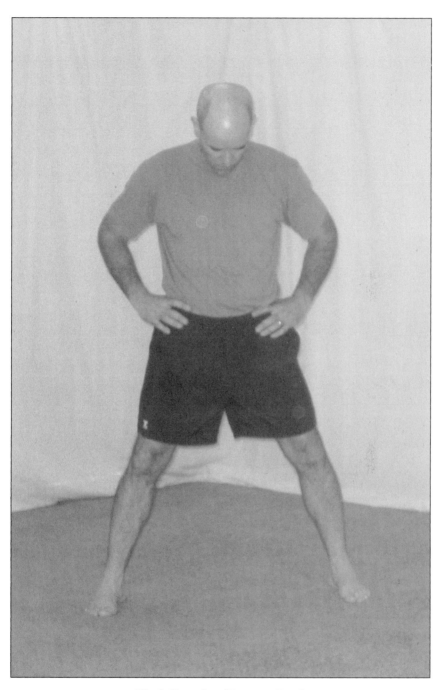

Neck Rotation Front to Back

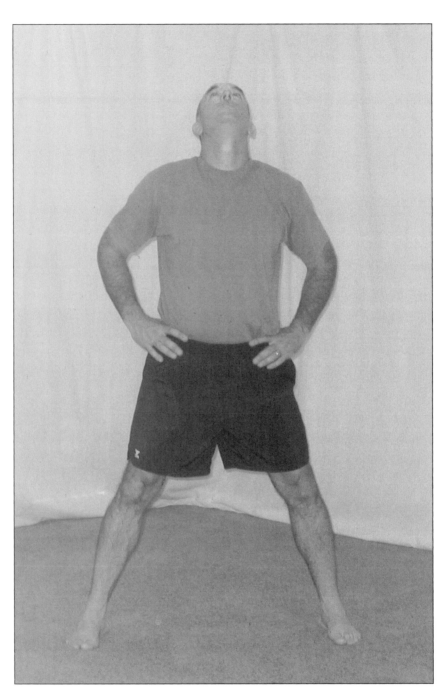

Neck Rotation Front to Back

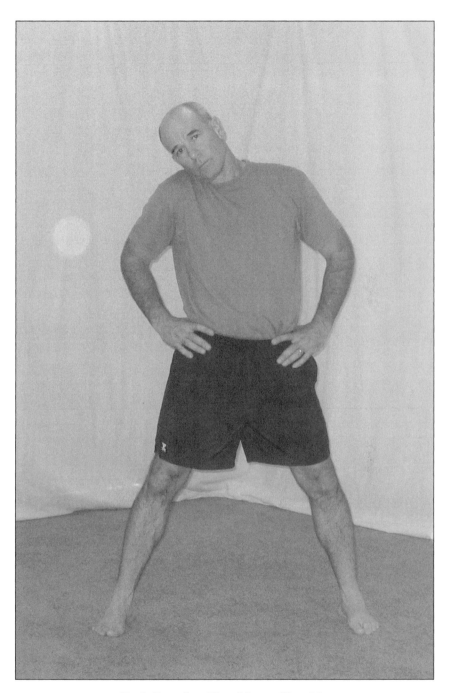

Neck Rotation Shoulder to Shoulder

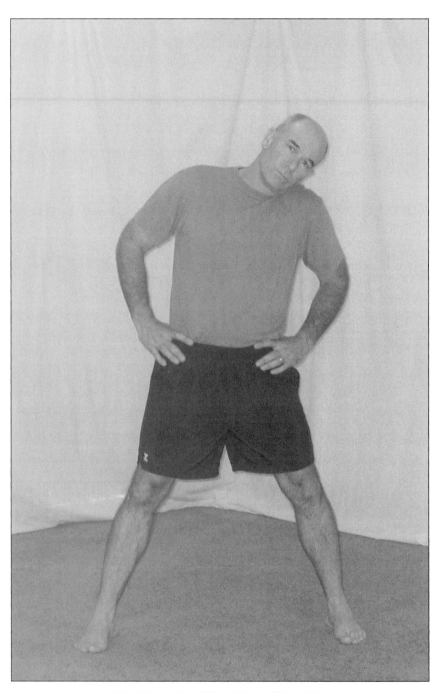

Neck Rotation Shoulder to Shoulder

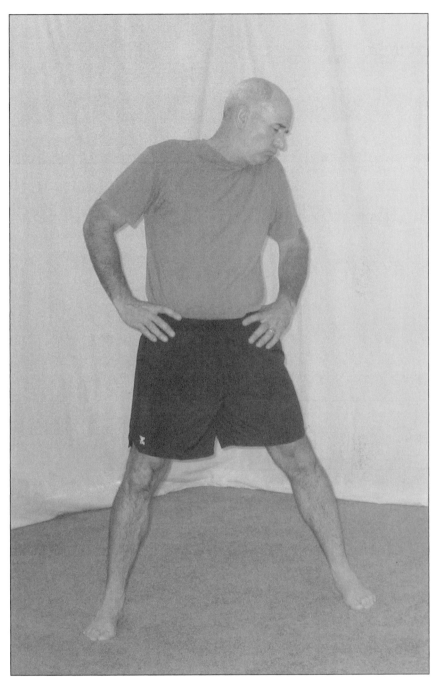

Neck Rotation 360 Degrees

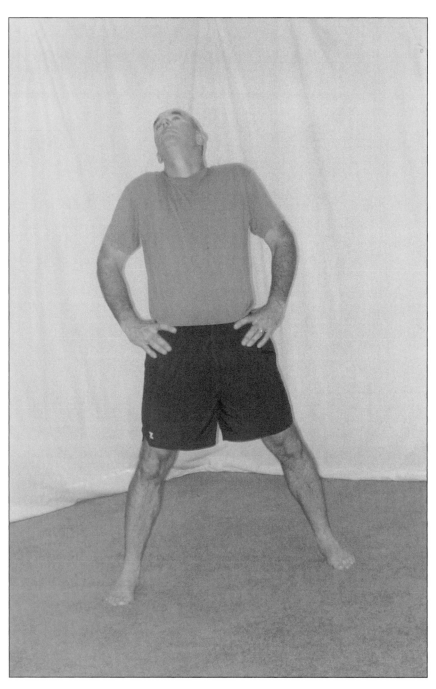

Neck Rotation 360 Degrees

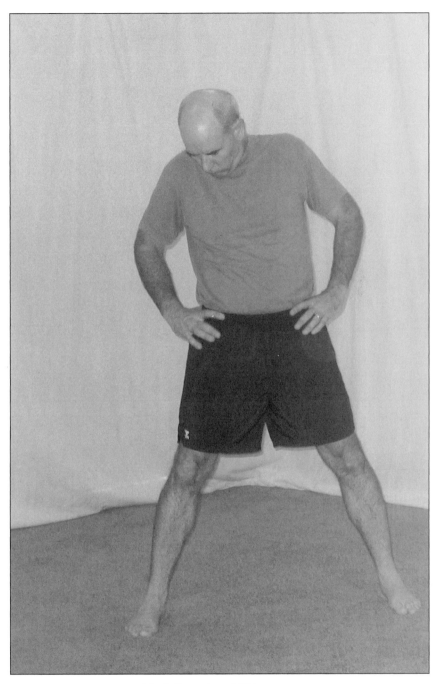

Neck Rotation 360 Degrees

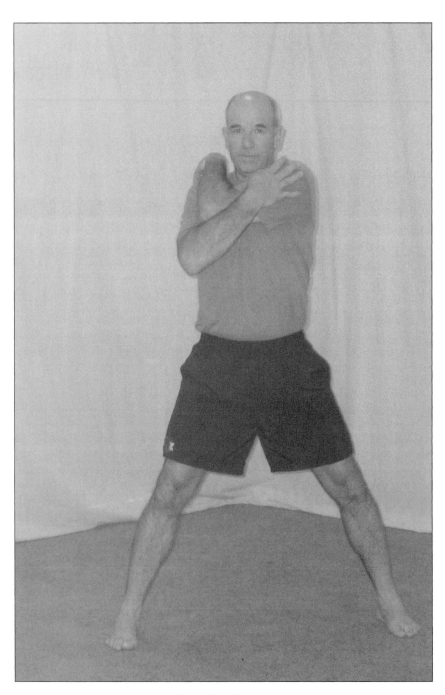

Shoulder Stretch

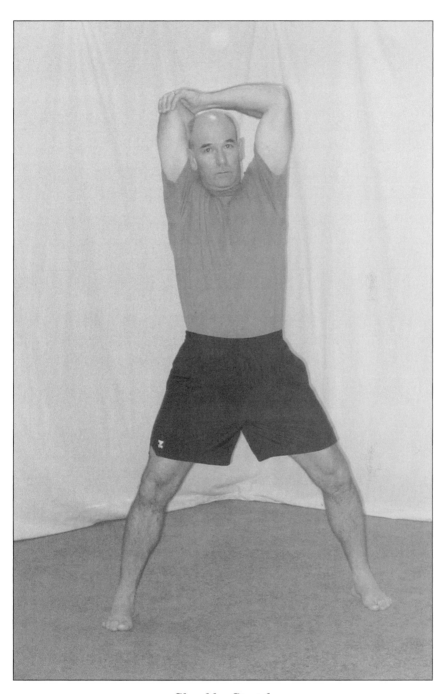

Shoulder Stretch

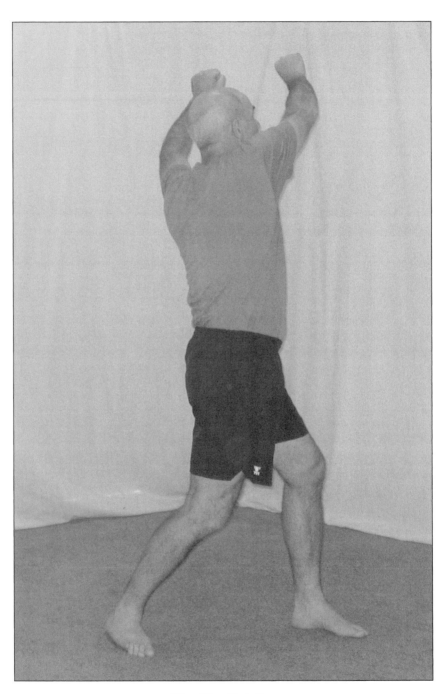

Shoulder Rotation

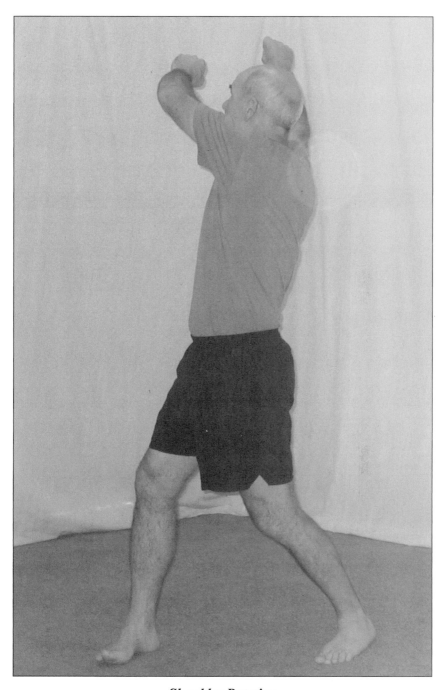

Shoulder Rotation

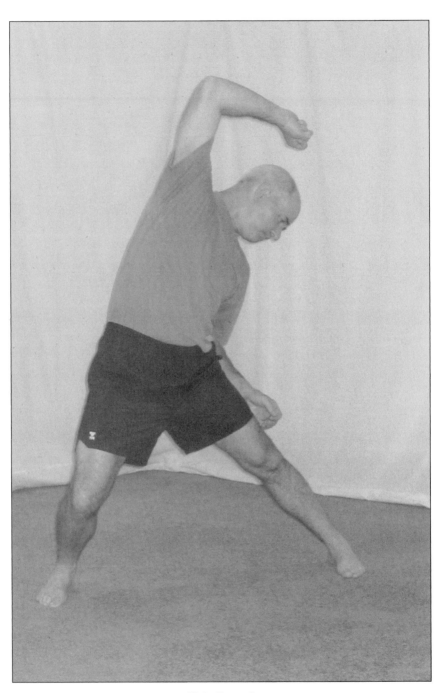

Side Stretch

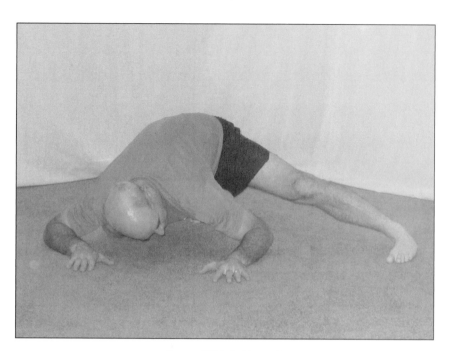

Inner Thigh Stretch

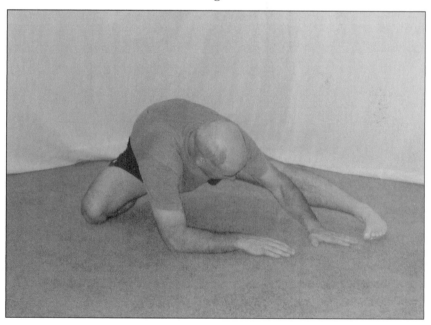

Inner Thigh Stretch

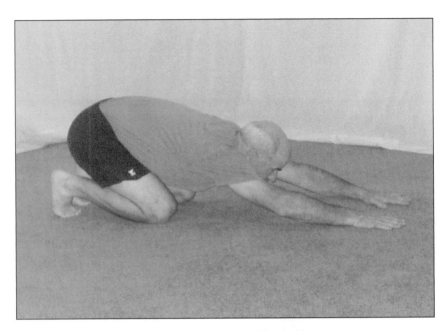

Toe and Shoulder Stretch

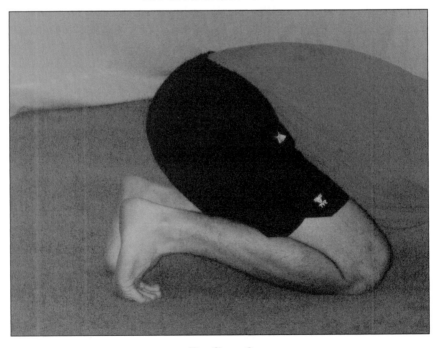

Toe Stretch

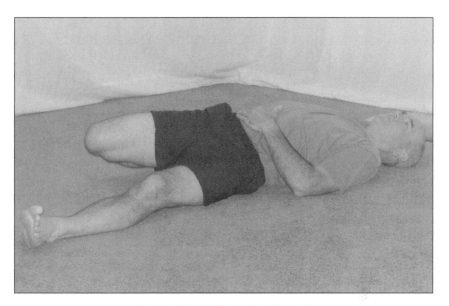

Front Thigh/Shoulder Stretch

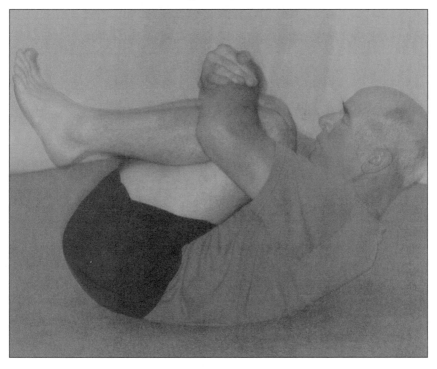

Lower Back Stretch

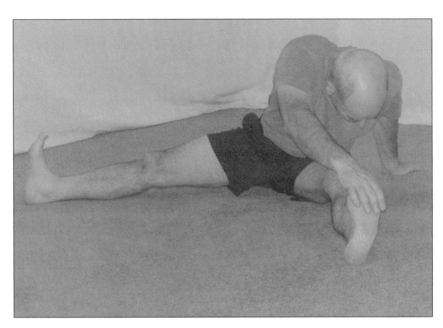

Combination Stretch

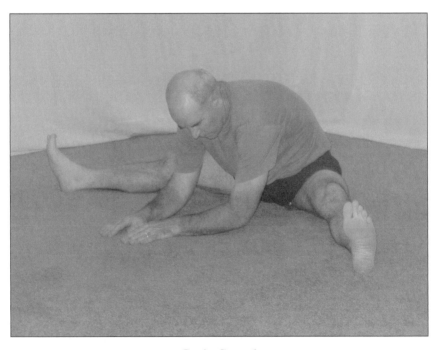

Groin Stretch

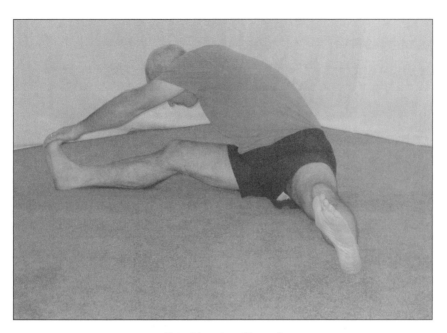

Combination Stretch

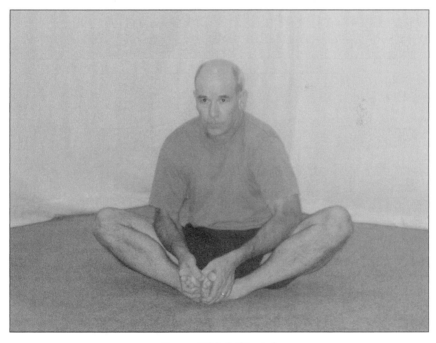

Inner Thigh Stretch

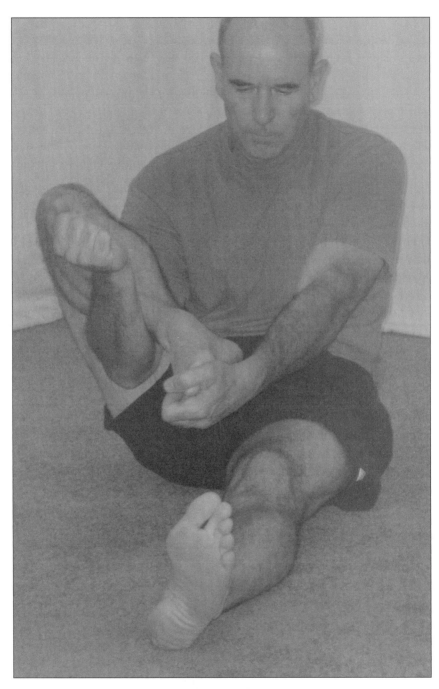

Ankle Rotations

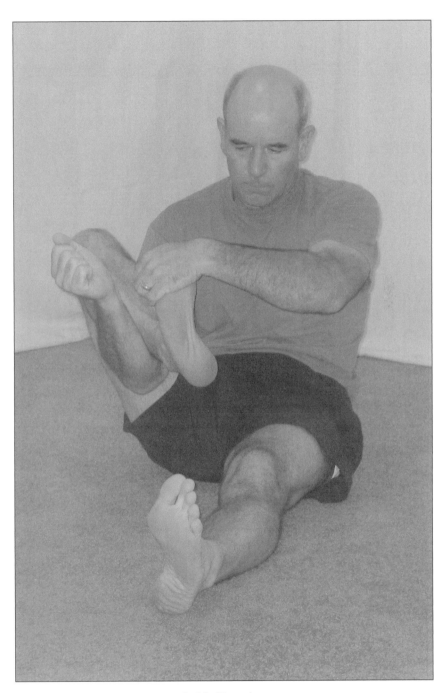

Ankle Rotations

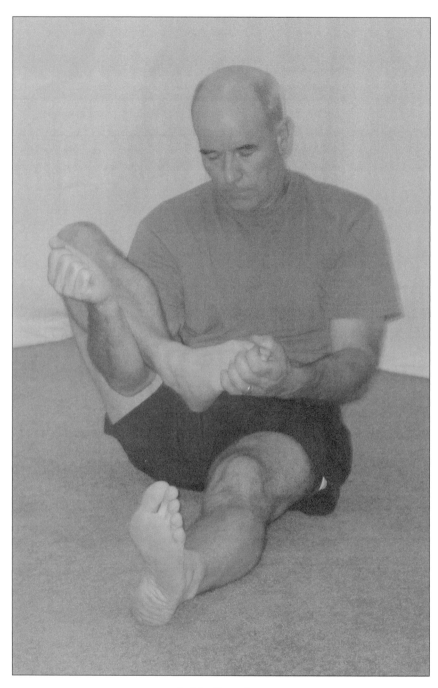

Ankle Rotations

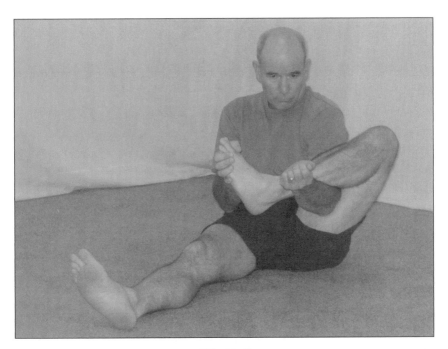

Hip Pull

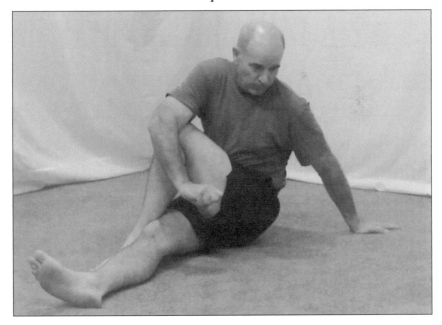

Glute Pull

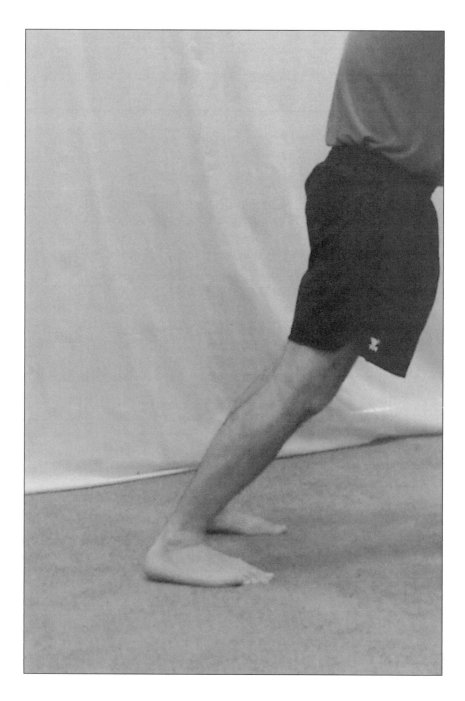

Calf Stretch

MUSCULAR STRENGTH AND CONDITIONING EXERCISES

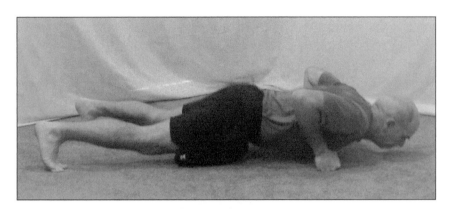

Knuckle Pushups

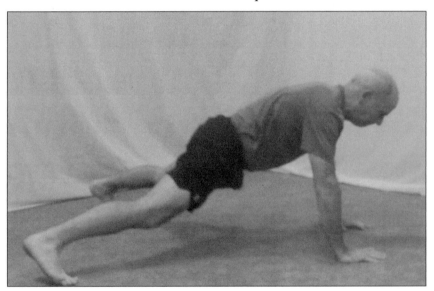

Chinese Pushup

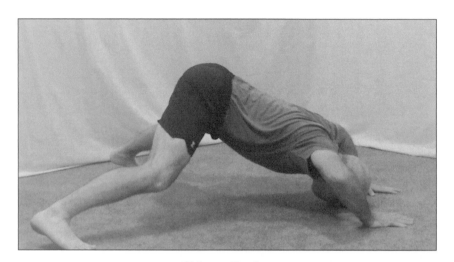

Chinese Pushup

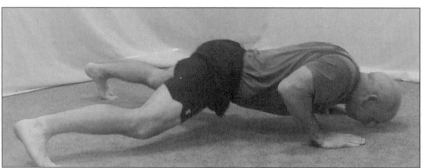

Chinese Pushup

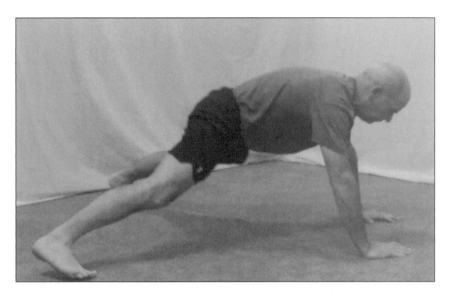

Chinese Pushup

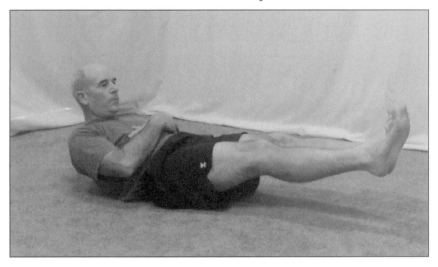

Ab Crunch/Leg Lift

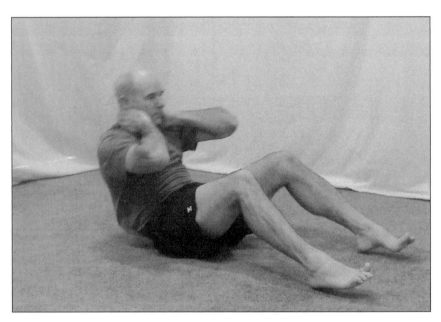

Ab Crunch/Sit Up

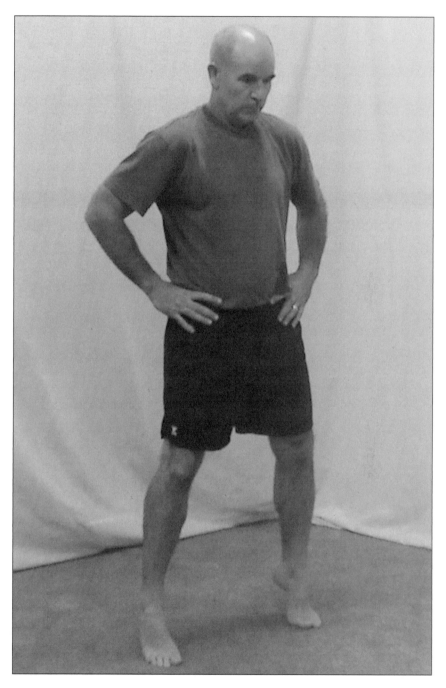

Ankle Lifts

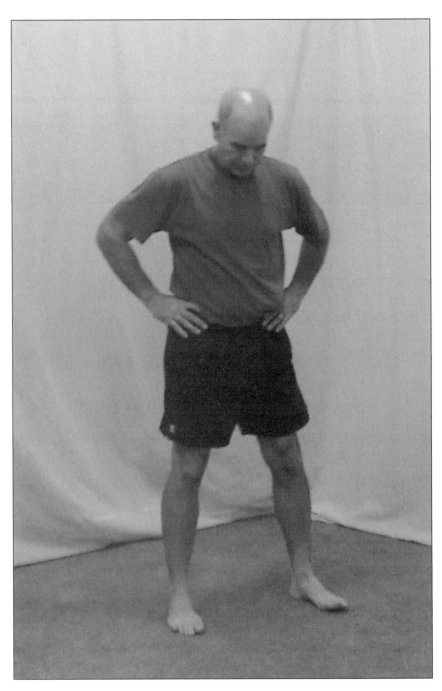

Ankle Lifts

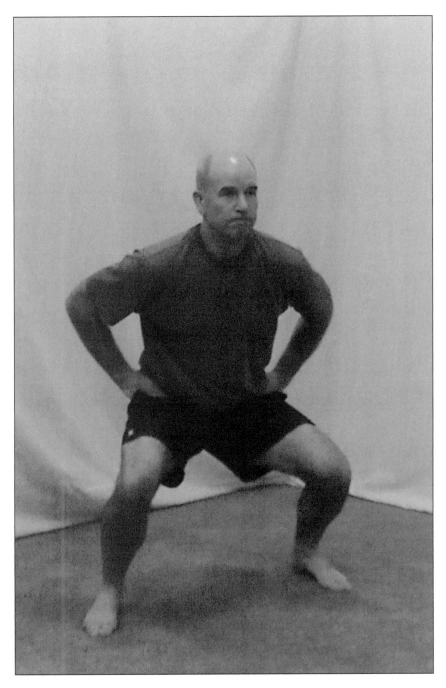

Squats

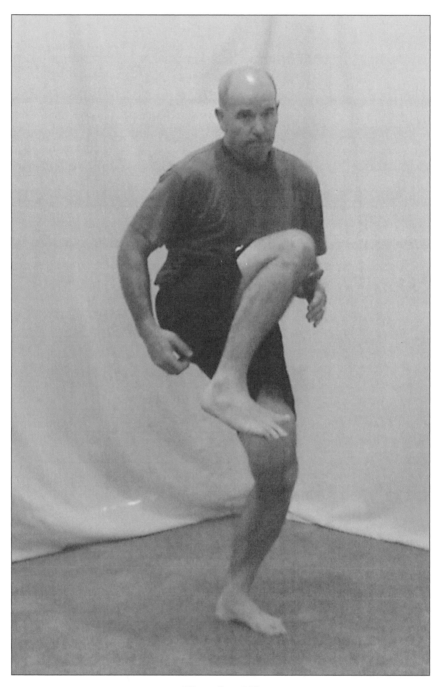

Chamber Lift

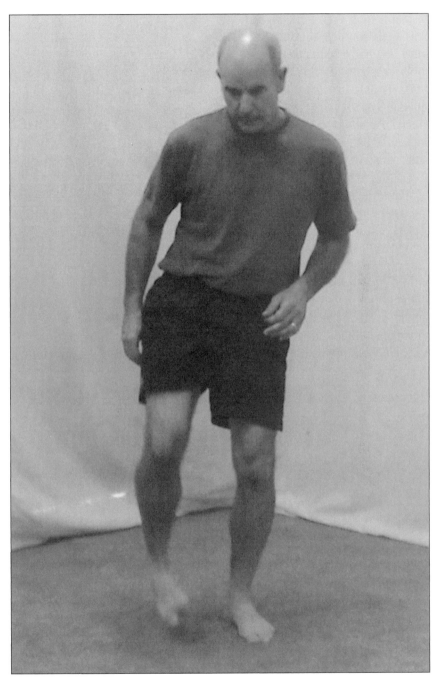

Side Lift

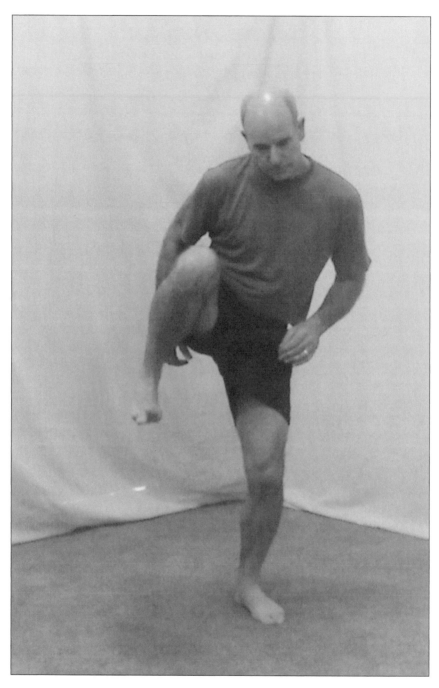

Side Lift

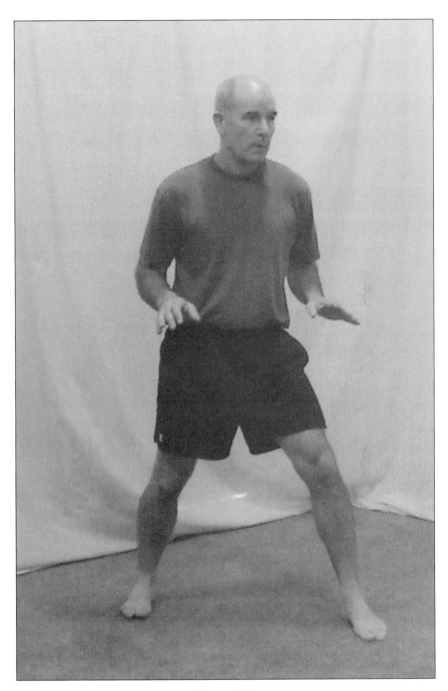

Front Lift

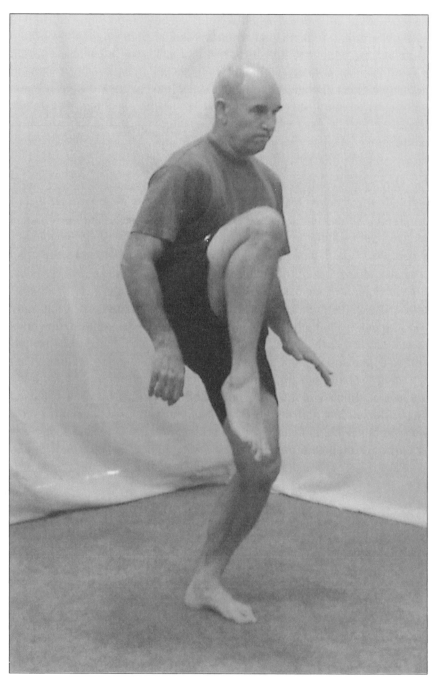

Front Lift

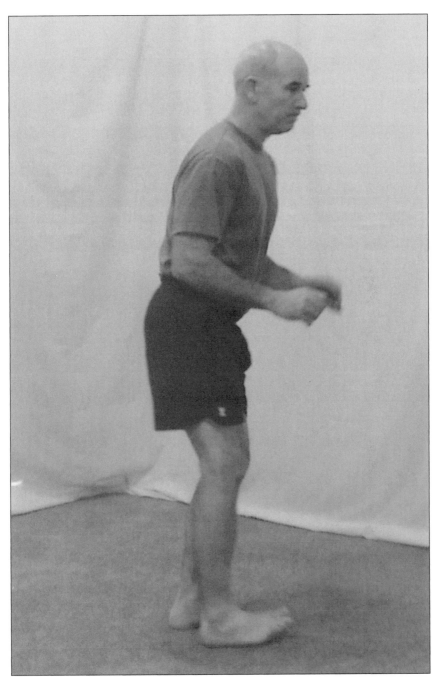

Rear Lift

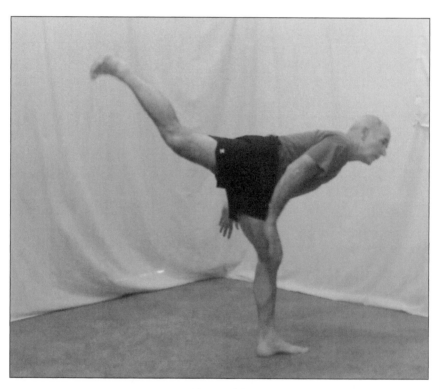

Rear Lift

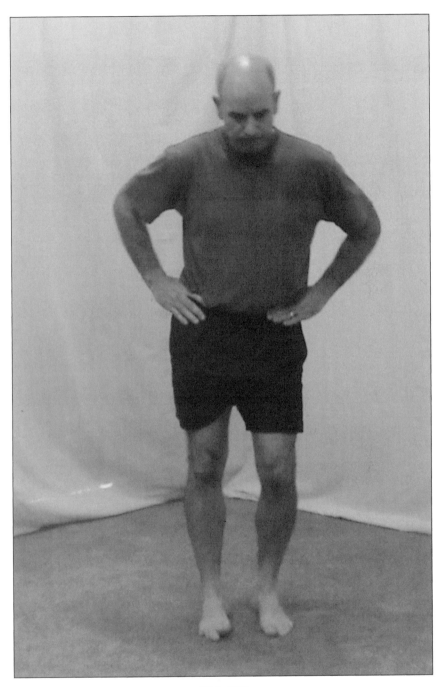

Side Lift

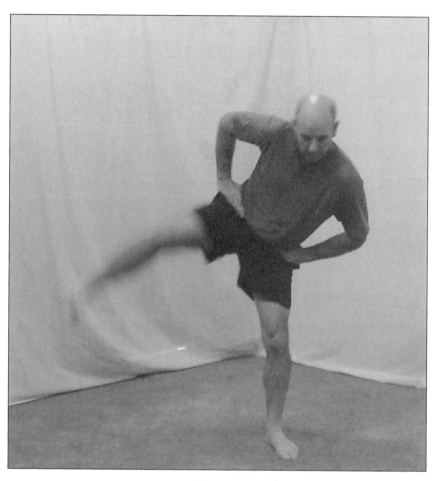

Side Lift

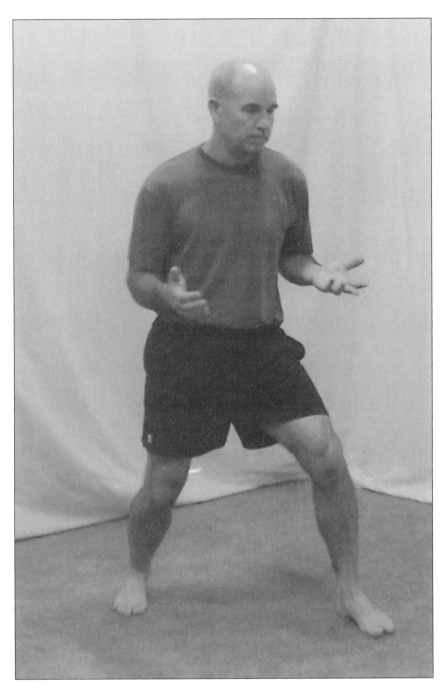

Front Lift

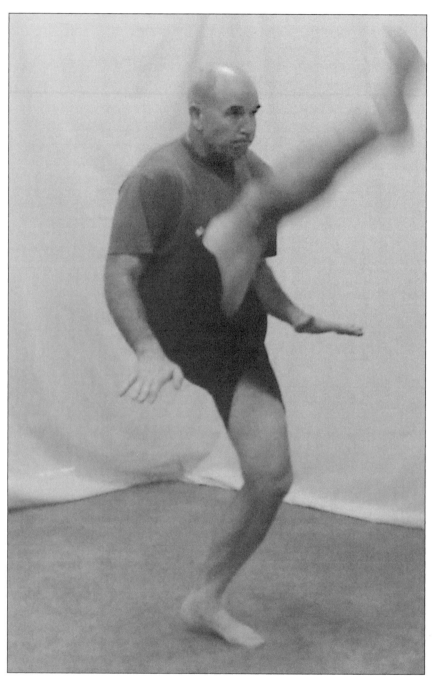

Front Lift

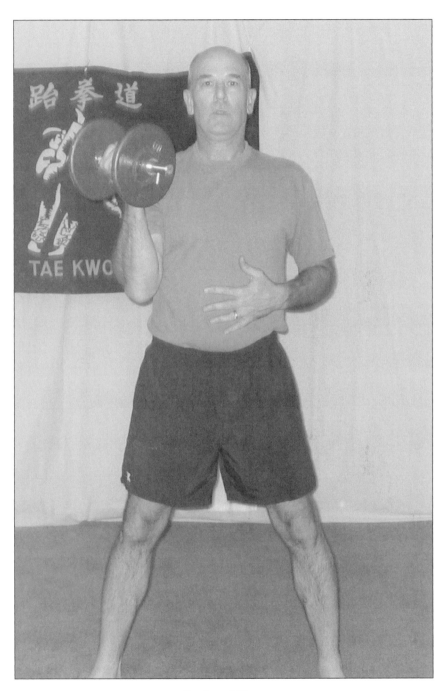

Curl and Press

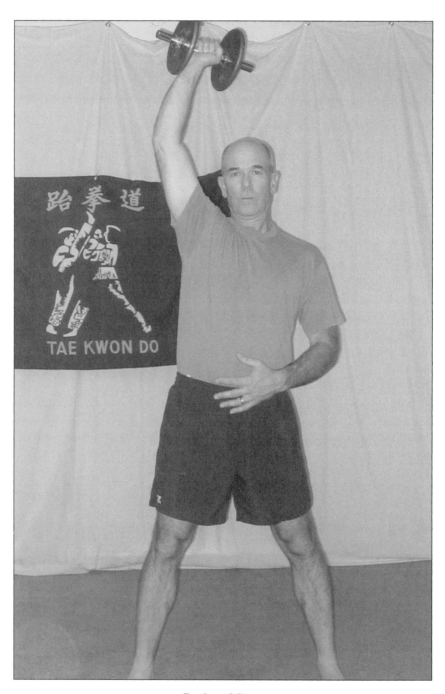

Curl and Press

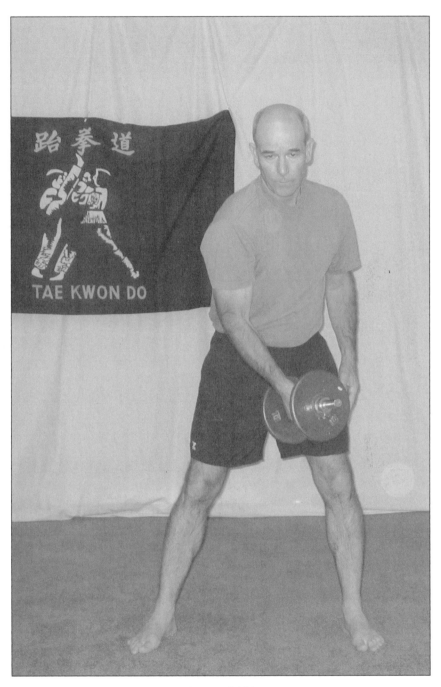

Lateral Lift

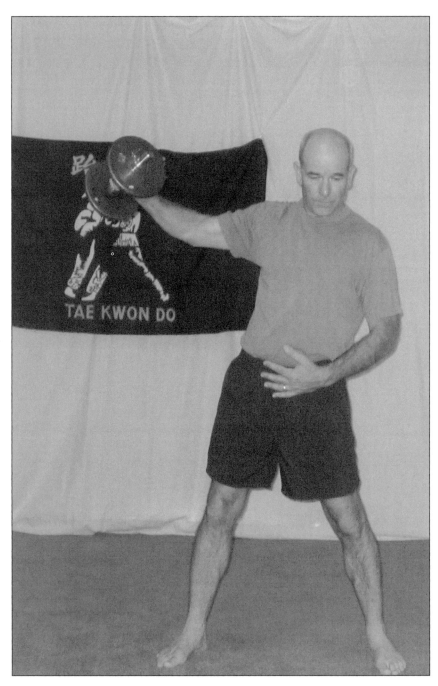

Lateral Lift

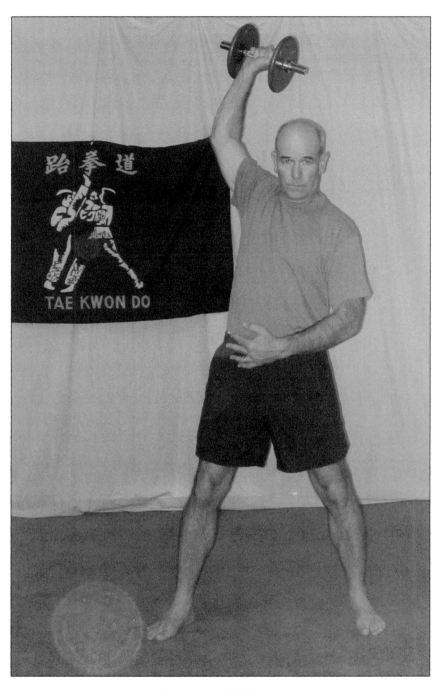

Lateral Lift

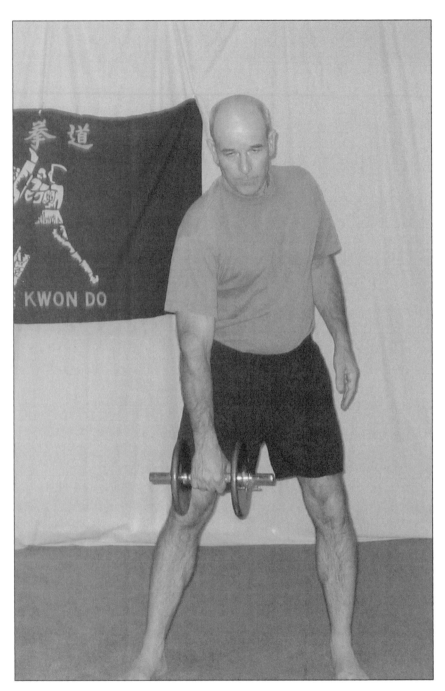

Shoulder Shrug

Shoulder Shrug

About the Author

Dr Brian Bolstad is a typical General Dentist, engaged in private practice in Sacramento, California. With a family and a house, he deals with the same demands on his time as do you. He has the same problems finding time to work out and train. He resumed his training in Martial arts at the age of 49 after a 30 year hiatus. Now at 52, he is currently working on a second degree Black Belt in Kenpo and a first degree Black Belt in Arnis. He is not an exeptional human athletic specimen and is a firm believer that you can do this too.

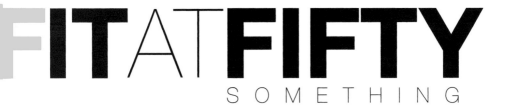

FIT AT FIFTY
SOMETHING

Order your workout DVD through the website at

fitatfiftysomething.com

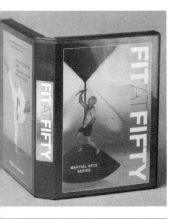

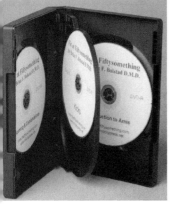

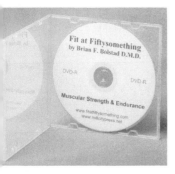

There are a total of six dvds - two single dvds and one set of four dvds.

Single DVDs - $14.95 each

- Flexibility and Range of Motion
- Muscular Strength and Endurance

Four Disk Set - $49.95

- The Martial Arts Series"

The individual disks in the Martial Arts Series:

- Fundamentals of Karate
- Kicks
- Sparring and Combinations
- Introduction to Arnis